First Printing Edition, 2021

ISBN: 9798598291375

Printed in the United Stated of America

Available from Amazon.com and Other Retail Outlets

Copyright © 2021 By Taahira Maskwa

All Right Reserved

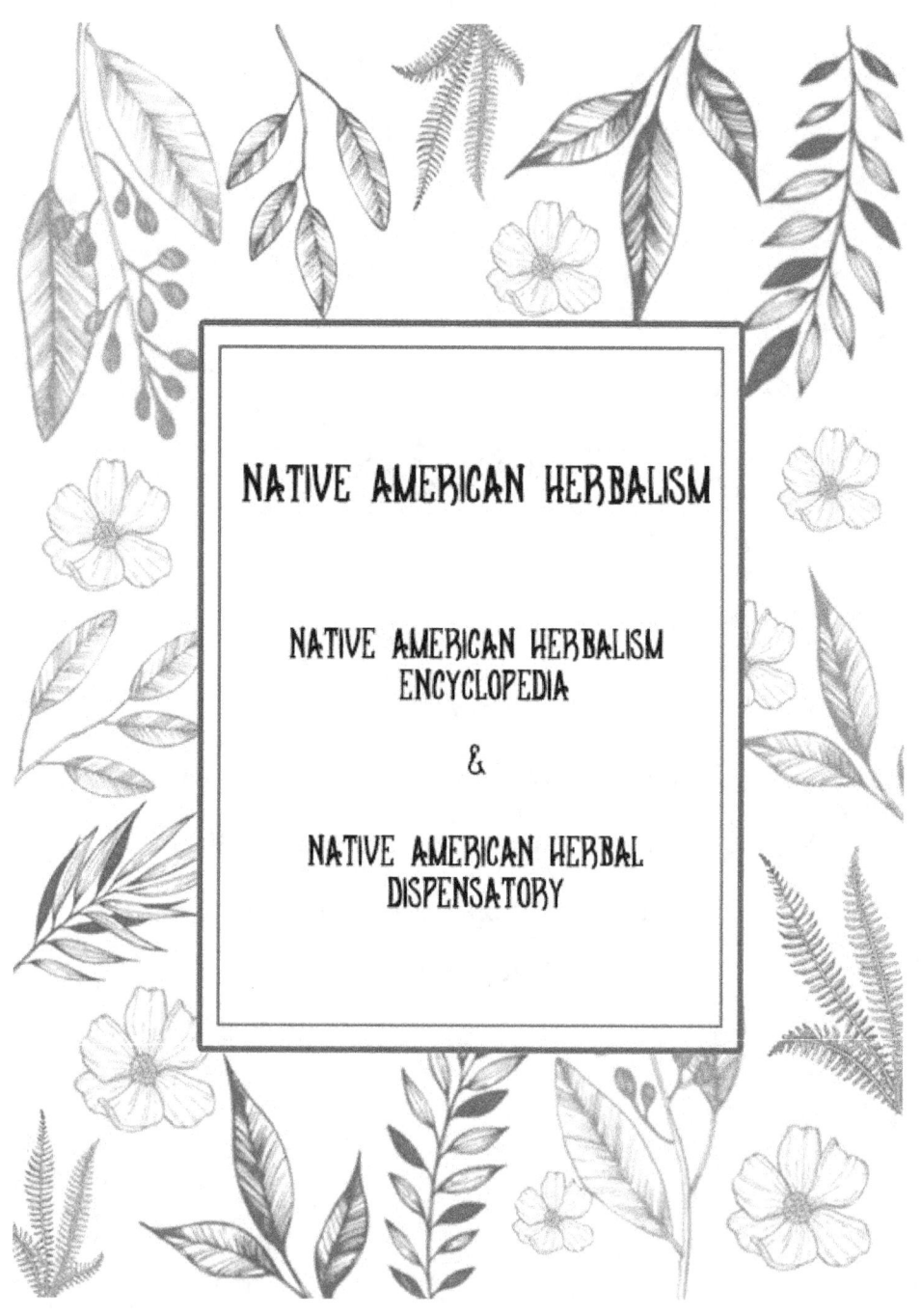

NATIVE AMERICAN HERBALISM

NATIVE AMERICAN HERBALISM ENCYCLOPEDIA

&

NATIVE AMERICAN HERBAL DISPENSATORY

TABLE OF CONTENTS

NATIVE AMERICAN HERBALISM ENCYCLOPEDIA 7
INTRODUCTION 8
    Native American Cultures 9
CHAPTER 1 : NATIVE AMERICAN MEDICINE AND MODERN USES 19
    Treatment Approaches - Different Types Of Treatments 20
    Short Summary Of Native American Medicine 21
    Native American Herbal Medicine And Modern Health Supplements . 28
CHAPTER 2 : MEDICINAL PLANTS 32
    Wildcrafting 34
    Tips For Wildcrafting Medicinal Herbs 34
    Growing And Propagation 38
    Collecting, Drying, And Storing Medicinal Plants 43
    6 Tips For Storing Dried Herbs 45
    Here Is A Good List To Follow When Labeling: 47
    Herbal Preparation Methods 48
    Decoction 49
    Juice 50
    Fomentation 50
    Poultice 51
    Ointment / Salve 53

Tincture / Liniment 54

Macerations 56

Syrup 57

Powder / Capsules 58

Pills / Lozenge / Suppository 58

Importance of Medicinal Plants And Herbs 60

Importance of Some Herbs With Their Medicinal Values 61

Misuse of Medicinal Plants And Herbs 63

Tips For Using Medicinal Herbs Safely 64

Essential Tools And Useful Instruments 65

CHAPTER 3 : NATIVE AMERICAN HERBS 69

1. Aloe - Aloe Doctrina 69

2. Arsesmart - Polygonum Hydropiper 76

4. Black Root - Veronicastrum Virgin Icum 82

5. Black Walnut - Juglans Nigra 85

6. Bloodroot - Sanguinaria Canadensis 89

7. Bearberry - Uva Urst 92

8. Capsicum - Capsicum Minimum, C. Frutescens 94

9. Catnip - Nepeta Cataria 97

10. Chamomile - Chamaemelum Nobile 98

11. Centaury - Centaurium Ervtraea 99

12. Chaga - Inonotus Obliquus 102

13. Chickweed - Stellaria Media 104

14. Damiana - Turnera Dif Usa Var. Aphrodisiac 105

15. Dandelion - Taraxacum Of Icinale 108

16. Echinacea - Echinacea Angustifolia 113

17. Feverfew - Chrysanthemum Parthenium 119

18. Gravel Root - Eutrochium Purpureum 124

19. Hops - Humulus Lupulus 127

20. Mullein - Verbascum 130

21. Nettle - Urtica Dioica 132

22. Oregon Grape - Mahonia Aquifolium 137

23. Primrose (Evening) Oil - Oenothera Biennis 140

24. Purslane - Portulaca Oleracea 147

25. Passionflower - Passiflora Incarnata 152

26. Red Clover - Trifolium Pratense 156

27. Sassafras Sassafras Albidum 162

28. Skullcup Scutellaria Lateriflora 165

29. Turkey Corn Dicentra Canadensis 168

30. Valerian - Valeriana Officinalis 169

31. Wormwood - Artemisia Absinthium 176

32. Witch Hazel Hamamelis Virginiana 180

    CONCLUSION 185

NATIVE AMERICAN HERBAL DISPENSATORY 187

INTRODUCTION 188

CHAPTER 1 : NATIVE AMERICAN TRADITIONS 192

  Spirituality And Connection 194

  Healers 195

  Symbolic Healing 197

  Healing And Ceremony 198

  Healing Plants 201

  Native Hawaiian Medicinal Plants 202

  Tools Used In Native American Healing Ceremonies 203

CHAPTER 2: TRADITIONAL REMEDIES FOR COMMON AILMENTS 208

Native American Medicine Today 208
Traditional Medicine For 213
    Abscess 213
    Acne 214
    Allergies 214
    Anxiety 215
    Asthma 216
    Backache 218
    Boils 218
    Bronchial Infections/Problems 220
    Burns 222
    Cancer 224
    Cough 225
    Constipation 229
    Cramps 232
    Diabetes 233
    Diarrhea 235
    Dropsy 238
    Eye Problems, Irritation, Soreness 240
    Fever 241
    Flu 244
    Heartburn 247
    Infection 248
    Inflammation/Swelling 248
    Insect Bites And Stings 253
    Menstrual Cramps And Pain 254
    Pneumonia 255

- Stomach Problems 256
- Syphilis 257
- Wounds 258

CHAPTER 3: MOST COMMON DIY HERBAL RECIPES 261
- 1. Tea 261
- 2. Decoctions 264
- 3. Popsicles 265
- 4. Ice Cubes 268
- 5. Bath 269
- 6. Breast milk 270
- 7. Compresses 273
- 8. Poultice 275
- 9. Tinctures 277

CHAPTER 4: HERBAL REMEDIES FOR YOUR CHILD 282
- 0-2 Month 282
- 2-12 Months 288
- 12 Months-5 Years 295
- 5 years-12 years 297

CONCLUSION 302

NATIVE AMERICAN HERBALISM ENCYCLOPEDIA

A Complete Medical Handbook of Native American Herbs

Taahira Maskwa

INTRODUCTION

Native American cultures across the United States are notable for their wide variety and diversity of lifestyles, regalia, art forms, and beliefs. The culture of indigenous North America is usually defined by the concept of the Pre-Columbian culture area, namely a geographical region where shared cultural traits occur. The northwest culture area, for example, shared common traits such as salmon fishing, woodworking, large villages or towns, and a hierarchical social structure. Though cultural features, language, clothing, and customs vary enormously from one tribe to another, certain elements are encountered frequently and shared by many tribes. Early European American scholars described the Native Americans as having a society dominated by clans.

Native American Cultures

Many thousands of years before Christopher Columbus' ships landed in the Bahamas, a different group of people discovered America: the nomadic ancestors of modern Native Americans who hiked over a "land bridge" from Asia to what is now Alaska more than 12,000 years ago. In fact, by the time European adventurers arrived in the 15th century A.D., scholars estimate that more than 50 million people were already living in the Americas. Of these, some 10 million lived in the area that would become the United States. As time passed, these migrants and their descendants pushed south and east, adapting as they went. To keep track of these diverse groups, anthropologists and geographers have divided them into "culture areas," or

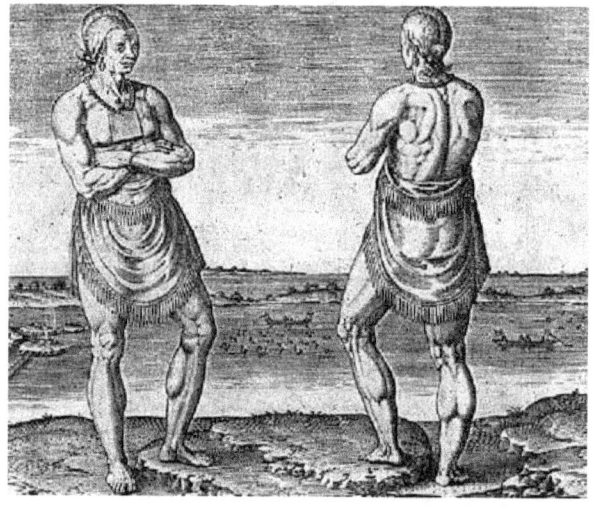

rough groupings of contiguous peoples who shared similar habitats and characteristics. Most scholars break North America excluding present-day Mexico into separate cultural areas: the Arctic, the Subarctic, the Northeast, the Southeast, the Plains, the Southwest, the Great Basin, California, the Northwest Coast, and the Plateau.

NATIVE AMERICAN CULTURAL REGIONS

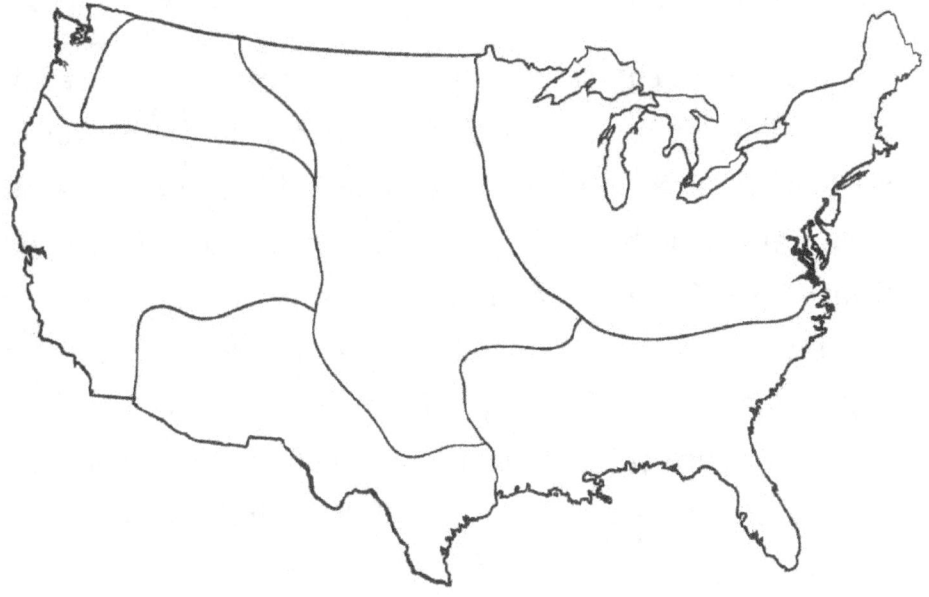

1. The Arctic

The Arctic culture area, a cold, flat, treeless region (actually a frozen desert) near the Arctic Circle in present-day Alaska,

Canada, and Greenland, was home to the Inuit and the Aleut. Both groups spoke, and continue to speak, dialects descended from what scholars call the Eskimo-Aleut language family. Because it is such an inhospitable landscape, the Arctic's population was comparatively small and scattered. Some of its peoples, especially the Inuit in the northern part of the region, were nomads, following seals, polar bears, and other game as they migrated across the tundra. In the southern part of the region, the Aleut were a bit more settled, living in small fishing villages along the shore.

The Inuit and Aleut had a great deal in common. Many lived in dome-shaped houses made of sod or timber (or, in the North, ice blocks). They used seal and otter skins to make warm, weatherproof clothing, aerodynamic dogsleds, and long, open fishing boats (kayaks in Inuit; baidarkas in Aleut). By the time the United States purchased Alaska in 1867, decades of oppression and exposure to European diseases had taken their toll: The native population had dropped to just 2,500; the descendants of these survivors still make their home in the area today.

2. The Subarctic

The Subarctic culture area, mostly composed of swampy, piney forests (taiga) and waterlogged tundra, stretched across much of inland Alaska and Canada. Scholars have divided the region's people into two language groups: the Athabaskan speakers at its western end, among them the Tsattine (Beaver), Gwich'in (or Kuchin) and the Deg Xinag (formerly and pejoratively known as the Ingalik), and the Algonquian speakers at its eastern end, including the Cree, the Ojibwa, and the Naskapi. In the Subarctic, travel was difficult toboggans, snowshoes and lightweight canoes were the primary means of transportation and the population was sparse. In general, the peoples of the Subarctic did not form large permanent settlements; instead, small family groups stuck together as they traipsed after herds of caribou. They lived in small, easy-to-move tents and lean-tos, and when it grew too cold to hunt they hunkered into underground dugouts.

3. The Northeast

The Northeast culture area, one of the first to have sustained contact with Europeans, stretched from present-day Canada's Atlantic coast to North Carolina and inland to the Mississippi River valley. Its inhabitants were members of two main groups: Iroquoian speakers (these included the Cayuga, Oneida, Erie, Onondaga, Seneca, and Tuscarora), most of whom lived along inland rivers and lakes in fortified, politically stable villages, and the more numerous Algonquian speakers (these included the Pequot, Fox, Shawnee, Wampanoag, Delaware, and Menominee) who lived in small farming and fishing villages along the ocean. There, they grew crops like corn, beans, and vegetables.

Life in the Northeast culture area was already fraught with conflict the Iroquoian groups tended to be rather aggressive and warlike, and bands and villages outside of their allied confederacies were never safe from their raids and it grew more complicated when European colonizers arrived. Colonial wars repeatedly forced the region's natives to take sides, pitting the Iroquois groups against their Algonquian neighbors. Meanwhile, as white settlement pressed westward, it eventually displaced both sets of indigenous people from their lands.

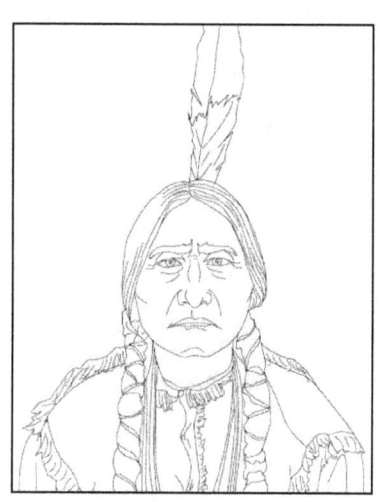

4. The Southeast

The Southeast culture area, north of the Gulf of Mexico and south of the Northeast, was a humid, fertile agricultural region. Many of its natives were expert farmers they grew staple crops like maize, beans, squash, tobacco, and sunflower who organized their lives around small ceremonial and market villages known as hamlets. Perhaps the most familiar of the Southeastern indigenous peoples are the Cherokee, Chickasaw, Choctaw, Creek, and Seminole sometimes called the Five Civilized Tribes, some of whom spoke a variant of the Muskogean language.

By the time the U.S. had won its independence from Britain, the Southeast culture area had already lost many of its native people to disease and displacement. In 1830, the federal Indian Removal Act compelled the relocation of what remained of the Five Civilized Tribes so that white settlers could have their land. Between 1830 and 1838, federal officials forced nearly 100,000 Indians out of the southern states and into "Indian Territory" (later Oklahoma) west of the Mississippi. The Cherokee called this frequently deadly trek the Trail of Tears.

5. The Plains

The Plains culture area comprises the vast prairie region between the Mississippi River and the Rocky Mountains, from present-day Canada to the Gulf of Mexico. Before the arrival of European traders and explorers, its inhabitant's speakers of Siouan, Algonquian, Caddoan, Uto-Aztecan, and Athabaskan languages were relatively settled hunters and farmers. After European contact, and especially after Spanish colonists brought horses to the region in the 18th century, the peoples of the Great Plains became much more nomadic. Groups like the Crow, Blackfeet, Cheyenne, Comanche, and Arapaho used horses to pursue great herds of buffalo across the prairie. The most common dwelling for these hunters was the cone-shaped teepee, a bison-skin tent that could be folded up and carried anywhere. Plains Indians are also known for their elaborately feathered war bonnets.

As white traders and settlers moved west across the Plains region, they brought many damaging things with them: commercial goods, like knives and kettles, which native people came to depend on; guns; and disease. By the end of the 19th century, white sport hunters had nearly exterminated the area's buffalo herds. With settlers encroaching on their lands and no way to make money, the Plains natives were forced onto government reservations.

6. The Southwest

The peoples of the Southwest culture area, a huge desert region in present-day Arizona and New Mexico (along with parts of Colorado, Utah, Texas, and Mexico) developed two distinct ways of life. Sedentary farmers such as the Hopi, the Zuni, the Yaqui, and the Yuma grew crops like corn, beans, and squash. Many lived in permanent settlements, known as pueblos, built of stone and adobe. These pueblos featured great multistory dwellings that resembled apartment houses. At their centers, many of these villages also had large ceremonial pit houses or kivas.

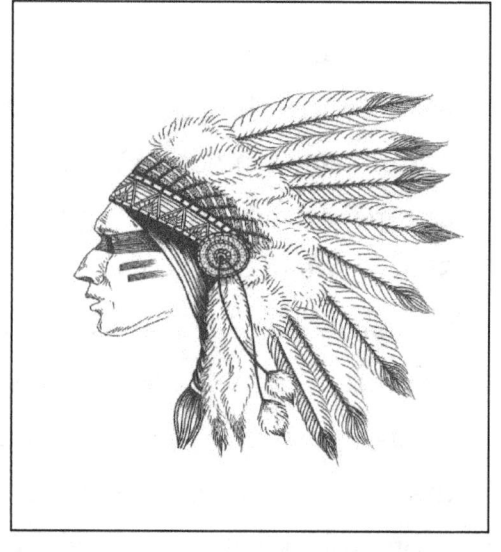

Other Southwestern peoples, such as the Navajo and the Apache, were more nomadic. They survived by hunting, gathering, and raiding their more established neighbors for their crops. Because these groups were always on the move, their homes were much less permanent than the pueblos. For instance, the Navajo fashioned their iconic eastward-facing round houses, known as hogans, out of materials like mud and bark.

By the time the southwestern territories became a part of the United States after the Mexican War, many of the region's native people had already been exterminated. (Spanish colonists and missionaries had enslaved many of the Pueblo Indians, for example, working them to death on vast Spanish ranches known as encomiendas.) During the second half of the 19th century, the federal government resettled most of the region's remaining natives onto reservations.

7. The Great Basin

The Great Basin culture area, an expansive bowl formed by the Rocky Mountains to the east, the Sierra Nevadas to the west, the Columbia Plateau to the north, and the Colorado Plateau to the south, was a barren wasteland of deserts, salt flats, and brackish lakes. Its people, most of whom spoke Shoshonean or Uto-Aztecan dialects (the Bannock, Paiute, and Ute, for example), foraged for roots, seeds, and nuts and hunted snakes, lizards, and small mammals. Because they were always on the move, they lived in compact, easy-to-build wikiups made of willow poles or saplings, leaves, and brush. Their settlements and social groups were impermanent, and communal leadership (what little there was) was informal.

After European contact, some Great Basin groups got horses and formed equestrian hunting and raiding bands that were similar to the ones we associate with the Great Plains natives. After white prospectors discovered gold and silver in the region in the mid-19th century, most of the Great Basin's people lost their land and, frequently, their lives.

8. California

Before European contact, the temperate, hospitable California culture area had more people an estimated 300,000 in the mid-16th century than any other. It was also more diverse: Its estimated 100 different tribes and groups spoke more than 200 dialects. (These languages derived from the Penutian (the Maidu, Miwok, and Yokuts), the Hokan (the Chumash, Pomo, Salinas, and Shasta), the Uto-Aztecan (the Tubabulabal, Serrano and Kinatemuk; also, many of the "Mission Indians" who had been driven out of the Southwest by Spanish colonization spoke Uto-Aztecan dialects) and Athapaskan (the Hupa, among others). As one scholar has pointed out, California's linguistic landscape was more complex than that of Europe.

Despite this great diversity, many native Californians lived very similar lives. They did not practice much agriculture. Instead, they organized themselves into small, family-based bands of hunter-gatherers known as tribelets. Inter-tribelet relationships, based on well-established systems of trade and common rights, were generally peaceful.

Spanish explorers infiltrated the California region in the middle of the 16th century. In 1769, the cleric Junipero Serra established a mission at San Diego, inaugurating a particularly brutal period in which forced labor, disease, and assimilation nearly exterminated the culture area's native population.

9. The Northwest Coast

The Northwest Coast culture area, along the Pacific coast from British Columbia to the top of Northern California, has a mild climate and an abundance of natural resources. In particular, the ocean and the region's rivers provided almost everything its people needed salmon, especially, but also whales, sea otters, seals and fish, and shellfish of all kinds. As a result, unlike many other hunter-gatherers who struggled to eke out a living and were forced to follow animal herds from place to place, the Indians of the Pacific Northwest were secure enough to build permanent villages that housed hundreds of people apiece. Those villages operated according to a rigidly stratified social structure, more sophisticated than any outside of Mexico and Central America.

CHAPTER 1 : NATIVE AMERICAN MEDICINE AND MODERN USES

Native American medicine refers to the combined health practices of over 500 nations. The specific practices varied among tribes but all are based on the basic principle that man is part of nature and health is a matter of balance. The natural world drives when it's interrelationships are honored, nurtured, and kept in harmony. The natural world cannot be seen by the eye and is not involved in technology, but is experienced directly and intuitively. Just as one cannot measure the inner life of a human being, nature has compelling forces that need to be integrated for balance. Native medicine is 40,000 years old. Documentation has only now begun and has been limited to observations therefore is incomplete. Native medicine honors all creation and is not just an academic body of knowledge or technique. Native American elders usually do not share their knowledge for fear of exploitation. Native American medicine addresses the balance in the inner life and overt behavior. The body, mind, spirit, emotions, social group, and lifestyle are all taken into account.

A patient's choice and preferences are always honored to create harmony.

Each Native American healer has their approach and can include bodywork, bone setting, midwifery, naturopathy, hydrotherapy, and botanical and nutritional medicine. Ceremonial and ritual medicine are also included. Much of this has been lost as this undocumented living tradition has only survived through living practitioners. More Native Americans have become interested in preserving their culture and through this effort Native, American medicine is as fluid today as ever.

Treatment Approaches - Different Types Of Treatments

Native American medicine is a complete system that balances every sphere of one's life from their inner world to lifestyle and social connections. Native medicine believes the roots of any imbalance are in the spiritual world. The spiritual interventions are critical to the process of any treatment plan.

Treatment approaches are always specifically and uniquely designed for the patient including fees and prices. They include the process of negotiating a fee as part of the healing process. The healing Elder has the most healing power and when treatment fails the elder practitioner loses the reputation as a powerful healer. The client in need of healing makes an offer to the medical practitioner and waits to see if it is accepted. They never negotiate face-to-face. The client leaves the offering outside the healer's door and if it is still there in the morning it has not been accepted and one can go elsewhere. Once they both agree, treatment may begin with the behavioral prescription, for example, a commitment, a selfless act, making amends, or climbing a sacred mountain. Techniques include self-inquiry and discovery to identify whether a lifestyle modification, herbs, prayer, massage, a sweat lodge ceremony, or a vision quest are necessary. GNC has been researching Indian herbs for a long time and has created some well-known supplements. You can try some with GNC coupons.

Training

Native American healers train their students through apprenticeships. Many years of testing a student's intention and commitment are essential for preparation. An apprentice learns patience, respect, and receives knowledge. Native medicine continues to be an oral tradition and cannot be learned in an academic setting. Only through experience can students learn the skills necessary and only when the student is ready does the elder teacher allow them to begin the practice of medicine.

Short Summary Of Native American Medicine

Many aspects of Native American healing have been kept secret and are not written down. The traditions are passed down by word of mouth from elders, from the spirits in vision quests, and through initiation. It is believed that sharing healing knowledge too readily or casually will weaken the spiritual power of the medicine.

There are, however, many Native American healers who recognize that writing down their healing practices is a way to preserve these traditions for future generations. Many also believe that sharing their healing ways and values may help all people to come into a healthier balance with nature and all forms of life.

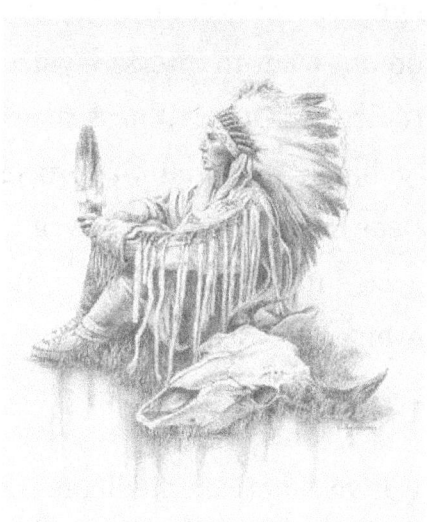

Benefits

Native American medicine can benefit anyone who sincerely wishes to live a life of wholeness and balance. These benefits may be physical, emotional, or spiritual. There is, however, the understanding that "the diseases of civilization," or white man's diseases, often need white man's medicine. In those cases, Native American medicine can be an important part of an integrative approach to healing. For example, the most successful programs for treating alcohol addiction in Native communities have combined Western approaches to psychological counseling, social work, and traditional Native American healing practices.

Such inherited conditions as birth defects or retardation are not easily treatable with Native American medicine. Native healers also believe that some illnesses are the result of a patient's behavior. Sometimes they will not treat a person because they do not want to interfere with the life lessons the patient needs to learn. Other illnesses are not treated because they are "callings" or initiation diseases. Native healer Medicine Grizzly Bear Lake explains, "The calling comes in the form of a dream, accident, sickness, injury, disease, near-death experience, or even actual death."

Description

Native American medicine is based upon a spiritual view of life. A healthy person is someone who has a sense of purpose and follows the guidance of the Great Spirit. This guidance is written upon the heart of every person. To be healthy, a person must be committed to a path of beauty, harmony, and balance. Gratitude, respect, and generosity are also considered to be essential for a healthy life. Ken Cohen writes, "Health means restoring the body, mind, and spirit to balance and wholeness: the balance of life energy in the body; the balance of ethical, reasonable, and just behavior; balanced relations within family and community; and harmonious relationships with nature."

Theories of disease causation and even the names of diseases vary from tribe to tribe. Diseases may be thought to have internal or external causes or sometimes both. According to Cherokee medicine man Rolling Thunder, negative thinking is the most important internal cause of disease. Negative thinking includes not only negative thoughts about oneself but also feelings of shame, blame, low self-esteem, greed, despair, worry, depression, anger, jealousy, and self-centeredness. Johnny Moses, a Nootka healer, says "No evil sorcerer can do as much harm to you as you can do to yourself."

Diseases have external causes too. "Germs are also spirits," according to Shabari Bird of the Lakota Nation. A person is particularly susceptible to harmful germs if they live an imbalanced life, have a weak constitution, engage in negative thinking, or are under a lot of stress. Other people or spirits may also be responsible for an illness. Another external source of the disease is environmental poisons. These poisons include alcohol, impure air, water, and some types of food.

Native American healers believe that disease can also be caused by physical, emotional, or spiritual trauma. These traumas can lead to mental and emotional distress, loss of soul, or loss of spiritual power. In these cases, the healer must use ritual and other ways to physically return the soul and power to the patient. Some diseases are caused when people break the "rules for living." These rules may include ways of showing respect for animals, people, places, ritual objects, events, or spirits.

Native American healers have several different techniques for diagnosing an illness. These may include a discussion of one's symptoms, personal and family history, observation of non-verbal cues like posture or tone of voice, and medical divination. More important than the particular technique is the healer's intuition, sensitivity, and spiritual power.

There is no typical Native American healing session. Methods of healing include prayer, chanting, music, smudging (burning sage or aromatic woods), herbs, laying-on of hands, massage, counseling, imagery, fasting, harmonizing with nature, dreaming, sweat lodges, taking hallucinogens (e.g., peyote), developing inner silence, going on a shamanic journey, and ceremony. Family and community are also important in many healing sessions. Sometimes healing happens quickly. Sometimes a long period is needed for healing. The intensity of the therapy is considered to be more important than the length of time required. Even if the healing happens quickly, however, a lifestyle change is usually required to make the healing last.

A medicine bundle may also be used in Native American healing. The medicine bundle is a bag made of leather or an animal pelt in which the healer carries an assortment of ritual objects, charms, herbs, stones, and other healing paraphernalia. The bundle is a concrete token of the medicine power that the spirits have given the healer, either for healing in general or for healing a particular illness. The bundles vary according to the clan, tribe, and individual.

Native American medicine is not covered by insurance unless perhaps the practitioner is a licensed health care provider. Most Native healers do not charge a set fee for their services. Healing is considered to be "a gift from the Great Spirit." Gifts to the healer are welcomed, however. The offering of a gift "ensures the success of treatment because healing spirits appreciate the generosity." Gifts may include groceries, cloth, money, or another personal expression of respect and appreciation. Frequently the only gift that is required is a pouch of tobacco.

Preparations

The medicine person tells the patient what preparations are necessary before the healing ceremony.

Precautions

A medicine person is essential to ensure safe healing through Native American medicine. People with hypertension should watch themselves during a sweat lodge ceremony for a possible increase in blood pressure. People with asthma may have difficulty when sage or cedar is used in a ceremony.

Claustrophobic people may find the close, hot, dark environment of a sweat lodge overwhelming.

Side Effects

Some herbs may cause vomiting, nausea, or diarrhea. From the Native American point of view, these reactions are usually welcomed and considered a form of purging or cleansing of the physical body.

Research & General Acceptance

There has been no formal scientific research conducted on Native American healing practices. Medicine people do not write down their practices out of fear that they might be misused by people who are not trained in their sacred ways. The most prominent users of this form of medicine are Native Americans or others who want a spiritually-based approach to medicine.

Training & Certification

Native American medicine has been passed down by word of mouth for thousands of years. Healing power can come from one's ancestors, another healer, or through training and initiation. Generally, healers train under one primary mentor. Today, however, with the ease of long-distance travel and communication, many healers have several mentors. Training as a medicine person is a long process that requires strength, sacrifice, and patience. Denet Tsosie, a Navajo medicine man, said that it took him six years to learn one of the chants.

Native American Herbal Medicine And Modern Health Supplements

Herbals And Herbalists

For most of human history, people have relied on herbalism for at least some of their medicinal needs, and this remains true for more than half of the world's population in the twenty-first century. Much of our modern pharmacopeia also has its roots in the historical knowledge of medicinal plants.

What Are Herbs, Herbals, And Herbalists?

To botanists, herbs are plants that die back to the ground after flowering, but more generally, herbs are thought of as plants with medicinal, culinary (especially seasoning), or aromatic uses. Traditional herbals are compilations of information about medicinal plants, typically including plant names, descriptions, and illustrations, and information on medicinal uses. Herbals have been written for thousands of years and form an important historical record and scientific resource. Many plant medicines listed in older herbals are still used in some form, but some herbals, especially earlier ones, also contain much inaccurate information and plant lore.

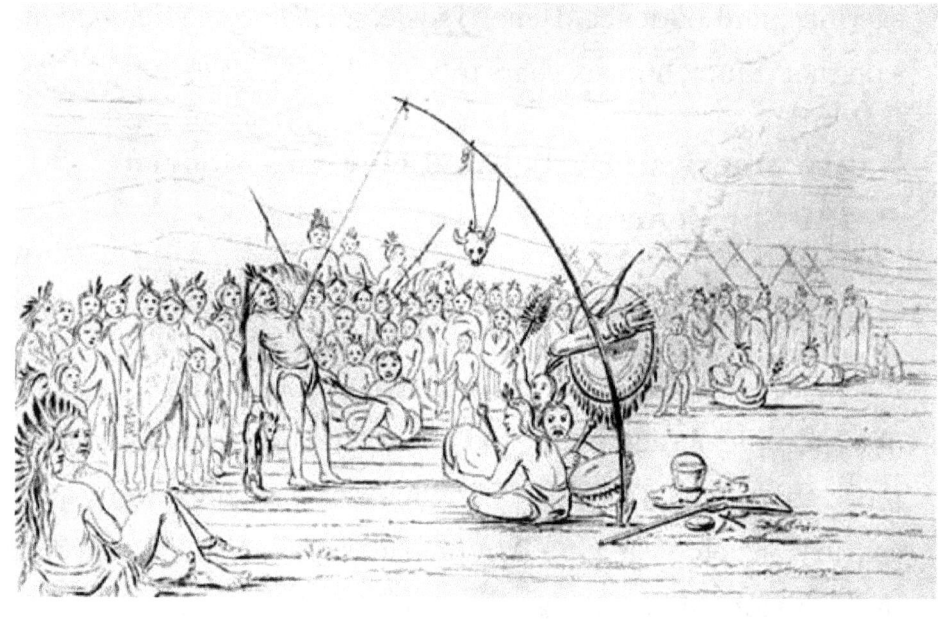

Herbalists follow a long tradition of using plants and plant-based medicines for healing purposes. Some gather medicinal plants locally, while others use both local and foreign plant material. Some rely on age-old knowledge and lore, while others also consult the findings of new research.

Herbal Medicine Today

Today, traditional herbalist healers continue to use the knowledge passed down for generations. Some ethnobotanists are studying with traditional healers to save such knowledge before it disappears. Due to a growing interest in alternative medicine, herbalism is also attracting new practitioners, and herbal research is constantly underway. Critics note that dosages can be difficult to control, even among plants of the same species, and side effects can be unpredictable.

Several essential modern drugs are derived from plants and scientists generally agree that only a fraction of the world's plants have been studied for their medicinal potential. However, threats to the environment, particularly in tropical forests where the highest numbers of species (many still unknown to science) reside, may reduce the possibility of identifying new plant-derived drugs.

How Plant Pharmaceuticals Are Discovered

The search for new pharmaceuticals from plants is possible using several distinct strategies. Random collecting of plants by field gathering is the simplest but least efficient way. The chances are much greater than new compounds of medicinal value will be discovered if there is some degree of selectivity employed by collecting those plants that a botanist knows are related to others already having useful or abundant classes of secondary metabolites. Even more relevant is to collect plants already targeted for specific medicinal purposes, possibly among indigenous or ethnic peoples who use traditional, plant-derived medicines often with great success to provide for their well-being. Such data are part of ethnobotany when researchers often obtain detailed information on the plants people use to treat illnesses, such as the species, specific disease being treated, plant part preferred, and how that part is prepared and used for treatment. This strategy can provide rapid access to plants already identified by traditional practitioners as having value for curing diseases, and this shortcut often sets the researcher rapidly on the road to the discovery of new drugs.

Taking the ethnobotanical approach, a specific part of the targeted ethnomedicinal plant is extracted, usually in a solvent like ethanol, and then studied in directed assays or tests to determine its value using, for instance, tissue-cultured cells impregnated with the organism known to cause the disease. For example, to assay for malaria the procedure could involve culturing red blood cells infected with the malarial-causing protozoan Plasmodium falciparum, placing a few drops of extract into the culture, and examining after a few days what effect, if any, the addition of the extract had on the protozoa. One final step in this process leading to the discovery of a new drug is to establish the mechanism of action of the compound, reactions in the body, and side effects or toxicity of taking it. The whole process from field discovery to a new pharmaceutical takes up to ten years and requires a multidisciplinary-interactive approach involving ethnobotanists, natural products chemists, pharmacognosists (those who study the biochemistry of natural products), and cell and molecular biologists.

CHAPTER 2 : MEDICINAL PLANTS

Plants can not run away from their enemies nor get rid of troublesome pests as humans or other animals do, so what have they evolved to protect themselves? Whatever this protection is it must be successful, for the diversity and richness of green plants is extraordinary, and their dominance in most ecosystems of the world is unquestioned. Plant successes are closely intertwined with the evolution and production of highly diverse compounds known as secondary metabolites, compounds that are not essential for growth and reproduction, but rather, through interaction with their environment, enhance plant prospects of survival. These metabolites are therefore planted agents for chemical warfare, allowing plants to ward off microorganisms, insects, and other animals acting as predators and pathogens. Such compounds may also be valuable to humans for the same purposes, and therefore may be used as medicines.

What Characterizes Medicinal Plants

There are twenty thousand known secondary plant metabolites, all exhibiting a remarkable array of organic compounds that provide a selective advantage to the producer, which outweighs their cost of production. Humans benefit from their production by using many of them for medicinal purposes to fight infections and diseases. An estimated two-fifths of all modern pharmaceutical products in the United States contain one or more naturally derived ingredients, the majority of which are secondary metabolites, such as alkaloids, glycosides, terpenes, steroids, and other classes grouped according to their physiological activity in humans or chemical structure.

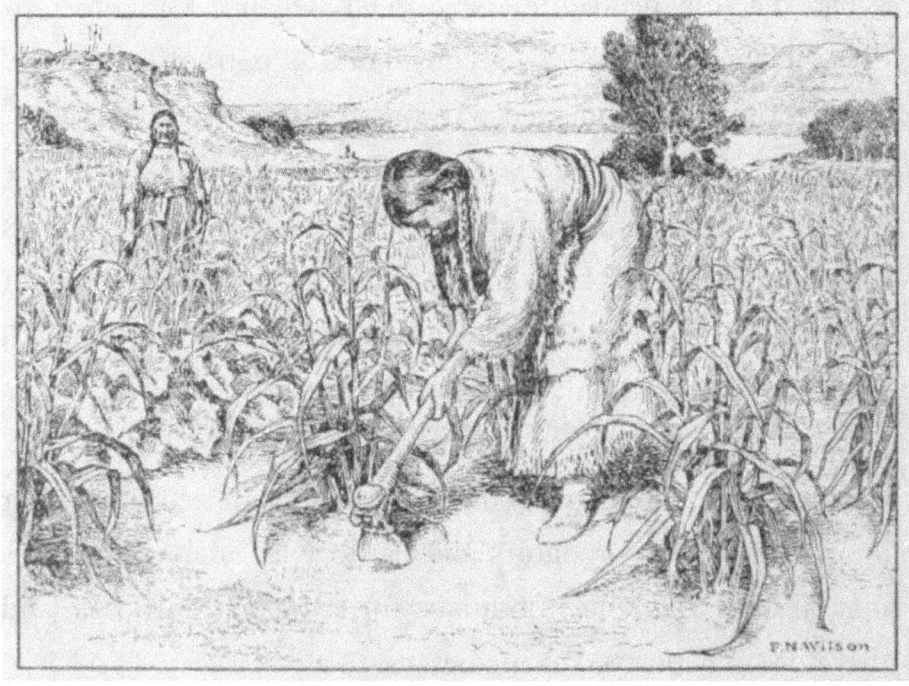

To illustrate the breadth of human reliance on medicinal plants, the accompanying table provides a list of the most significant plants, their uses in modern medicine, and the major secondary metabolites responsible for their activities. This list grows annually as new plants are found with desired activities and remedies to become pharmaceuticals for use in medicine.

Wildcrafting

Wildcrafting is the practice of foraging for useful plants from their natural, wild habitat for edible or medicinal purposes. It applies to uncultivated plants wherever they may be found, and is not necessarily limited to wilderness areas. Ethical considerations are often involved, such as protecting endangered species, the potential for depletion of commonly held resources, and in the context of private property, preventing theft of valuable plants, for example, ginseng.

Tips For Wildcrafting Medicinal Herbs

Here are 10 tips for wildcrafting medicinal herbs that will help you on your plant foraging journey.

1. **Get A Few Good Plant Identification Books For Your Area.**

You will want to invest in 2 or 3 good plant identification books to help you. It's especially helpful to find books that are geared towards medicinal and edible plants, and even better if you can find one specifically for your region. Try to go on a few plant walks with a local expert before venturing out on your own, and be 100% sure of your plant identification before harvesting, as there are some toxic lookalikes.

2. Be Prepared.

Before you leave, put together a backpack or bag with your plant books, water, a snack or two, extra clothing, and even a small first aid kit (make a Hiking First Aid Kit). You will also want to bring a pocket knife and scissors and/or small pruners for collecting. If you think you might be collecting some roots, a small gardener's trowel is also handy. Small baggies of some sort for your collections are helpful as well.

3. Get Outside!

This is the best part about wildcrafting, it gets you outside, exercising in nature, all with a purpose. It doesn't matter if you go for a long hike in the woods or a stroll in your neighborhood, medicinal plants grow everywhere. You just have to get outside and start looking!

4. Walk Slowly.

As a longtime hiker, this one was hard for me to start doing. I like to walk fast and get in some good mileage, but when your goal is to collect wild plants, you need to take it slow so that you have the chance to notice your surroundings. If you're like me and you have a hard time with slowing down, maybe take a child or an elderly person with you. They naturally walk slow and

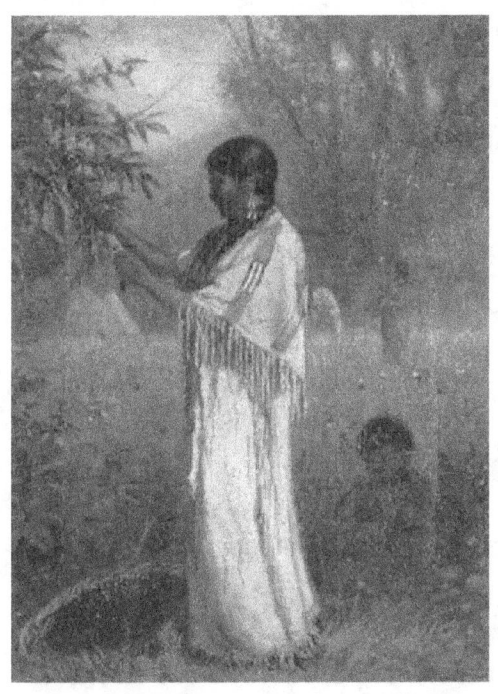

force you to move at a different pace, plus I'm sure they would love the adventure!

5. Keep Your Eyes Peeled.

As you're walking slowly, look down. Scan the trail, path, or sidewalk that you're walking on. Look in all directions, and sometimes even behind you. Look up. Stop from time to time just to take in your surroundings. Pick out plants and practice looking them up in your identification books. Just keep looking!

6. Look In Uncommon (And Common) Places.

When you're on the trail, try going off trail for a bit. Be gentle when doing this, as you don't want to disturb the natural habitat. Beyond the woods, however, there are many places to wildcraft.

Sidewalks and quiet gravel road edges are good places to look, as are open fields and empty lots. Make sure to get permission first for anything that is private property, and steer clear of busy roadsides to avoid runoff and pesticide contaminants. Also avoid areas that are close to industrial and construction sites, under power lines, or near commercial farms that could be using pesticides and have a toxic runoff. Many local places like parks, green spaces, and school grounds can also be good; just be sure to check that collecting wild plants is allowed before you start. Wherever you collect, be sure that the plants aren't being sprayed with pesticides and are not growing on polluted land, and always check if foraging is allowed. You might even want to look in your backyard!

7. Don't Set Out To Find A Specific Plant.

Unless you know without a doubt that a specific plant grows in a specific place, you don't want to set yourself up for failure by thinking that you're going to go out and collect a whole bunch of a certain plant. Half of the fun is the adventure and not knowing what you're going to find. Often, I will find several plant varieties, but on rare occasions, I won't find any. That's just how it goes sometimes.

8. Don't Overlook Common Plants.

There are so many medicinal plants that we have all grown up with that are easily identifiable. Dandelion, red clover, plantain, yarrow, mullein, rosehips, and elderberry are just a few. Learn about common plants like these first, then move on to more uncommon or harder to find plants.

9. **Be Mindful Of Plants That Are Rare Or Endangered.**

Research which medicinal plants are rare or endangered, and do not take any of those. Overharvesting can be devastating for many threatened plant species. Some examples of medicinal plants that are at-risk are slippery elm, American ginseng, black cohosh, and goldenseal.

10. **Leave More Than You Take.**

Finally, even for abundant plants, do not take them all. If you want these wonderful medicinal plants to keep on giving us their wonderful benefits, we have to leave some for future years. So always leave more than you take (a general rule is to harvest just 5-10% of a population), and better yet, plant a seed of the same variety whenever you remove a plant.

Wildcrafting is an endeavor that every herbalist should try. These 10 tips for wildcrafting medicinal herbs should give you a good head start. The most important part is to just start looking, soon you'll be surprised by how many plants you can identify!

Growing And Propagation

Medicinal plants can be cultivated by two methods (applicable to non-medicinal plants): Sexual and Asexual method

1. Sexual Method (Seed Propagation):

In this method, the plants are raised from seeds. Such plants are known as seedlings. Seeds are sown in the fields by methods like broadcast, dibbling, or placing them in drills or holes. The seeds must be of good quality, capable of high germination rate, and free from diseases.

Advantages:

- Seedlings are comparatively much cheaper and easy to raise.
- Seedlings are long-lived, bear more heavy fruits, and plants obtained are more sturdy.
- In those plants where other methods of cultivation cannot be utilized, seed propagation becomes the only method of choice.
- There are chances of production of some chance-seedlings of very high superiority which may be of great importance e.g., orange, papaya, etc.

Disadvantages:

- The seedlings obtained from this method require more time to bear and are not uniform in their growth and yielding capacity as compared to other methods like grafting.
- Also, the cost involved in harvesting and protection from pests is more.

2. Asexual Methods (Vegetative Propagation):

In this method, any of the vegetative parts of the plant like root or stem is provided such an environment that it develops into a new plant. The environment is provided by setting various parts of the plant in well-prepared soil.

1. Bulbs: A bulb is originally and structurally a bud, which possesses the capability of perennation. It consists of a very short stem ending in an apical meristem and enclosed by closely set leaves, which are thick and fleshy, being stored with reserves of food. Each of the leaves has of course its axillary bud.

After flowering, the foliage leaves persist for a time, forming food materials, which are now stored in one or more of the axillary buds. The axillary buds thus used as storehouses become the bulbs of the new generation. Whenever more than one new bulb is formed from an old one, there has been vegetative reproduction as well as perennation e.g., Squill, garlic.

2. Corms: In a corm, the storage organ is swollen base of the stem and this is wrapped in thin scale-leaves, each of which, of course, has an axillary bud e.g. colchicum, saffron.

3. Tubers: It is a swelling on an underground stem branch. The stem grows axillary buds formed low down on the aerial stem and push through the soil, swelling at their ends to form the tubers e.g., jalap, aconite, potato.

4. Rhizomes: In underground stems, the older parts of the rhizome die off. The buds borne on the detached younger portions thus become separate new plants e.g., ginger, turmeric.

5. Runners: The stem grows along the ground (horizontally over the surface of the soil), and produces roots and erect flowering shoots from lateral buds at many of its nodes. The growth of the creeping stem is continued by the terminal bud. Some of the older internodes die, and the detached rooted and shoot bearing parts become independent plants e.g., peppermint, strawberry.

6. Suckers: A shoot arising from a root of a woody plant e.g., mint, pineapple, banana.

7. Offsets: These originate from the axil of the leaf as short thick horizontal branches and are also characterized by the presence of rosette types of leaves and a cluster of roots at their bottom e.g., aloe, valerian.

8. Stolons: A creeping stem that roots at nodes e.g., arrow-root, licorice.

9. Cutting: A clear cut is made preferably below the node and the lower leaves are removed. It is then placed in a suitable medium and provided with suitable conditions of the moist atmosphere, temperature which favoring the development of roots e.g., mint, vanilla.

10. Layering: A layer is a branch or a shoot that is induced to develop roots before it is completely severed from the parent plant. It is done by a cut or ligature and embedding the part so treated in the soil e.g., cascara.

11. Grafting And Budding: Grafting is a process in which two cut surfaces of different but closely related plants are placed to unite and grow together. The rooted portion is called the stock and the cut-off is the scion or graft e.g., female scion of Myristica fragrans on the male stock to increase the fruit-bearing proportion.

12. Aseptic Methods Of Propagation: In this method, the plants are developed in an artificial medium under aseptic conditions from very fine pieces of plants like single cells, callus, seeds, embryos, root tips, shoot tips, pollen grains, etc. They are provided with nutritional and hormonal requirements.

Advantages (Asexual Method):

- ❖ There is no variation between the plant grown and the plant from which it is grown. As such, the plants are uniform in growth and yielding capacity.
- ❖ Seedless varieties of fruits can only be propagated vegetatively e.g., pomegranates, grapes, lemon.
- ❖ Plants start bearing earlier as compared to seedlings.

- Budding or grafting encourages disease-resistant varieties of plants.

Disadvantages:

- In comparison to seedling trees, these are not vigorous in growth and are not long-lived.
- No new varieties can be evolved by this method.

Collecting, Drying, And Storing Medicinal Plants

Drying Herbs

After you harvest your herbs, the next step is to preserve them in a way that prolongs their potency for future use. This allows us to have access to these medicinal herbs all year long. Drying (dehydrating) your herbs can be done in one of two easy ways at home.

Herbs dry best in warm, shaded, well-ventilated areas. It is not recommended to dry them in the sun; the intense heat and rays of the sun can quickly degrade the plant's medicinal constituents. Instead, I prefer to create small bundles of herbs that I hold together with a rubber band placed at the end of the stems. I then hang them upside down on a string in my kitchen window until they are dried completely. For each herb, the drying time will be different so check them daily. You may also choose to lay your herbs flat on a screen or oven rack placed on the counter. This way allows air to flow freely through the plant while they dry but it does take up valuable counter space for several days to a week.

If you have a food dehydrator, you can complete the drying process very quickly. You just set your dehydrator and be on your way.

If you are choosing to dry roots of herbs, I recommend that you clean and chop your roots while they are fresh, before drying. Once a root dries it may become so dense and tough that cutting it into small pieces could take an act of God. Doing some shopping ahead of time will save you a great deal of heartache.

Garbling Your Dried Herbs

Once you have completed the drying process, it is time to garble your herbs. Garbling is the process of separating the leaves, flowers, and stem portions and discarding the unwanted parts. Each medicinal herb has its medicinal part so be sure to research which part you are wanting from your chosen herb.

Storing Your Herbs

Once you have completed your drying and garbling it is time to store your herbs. For best preservation, you want to keep your herbs in airtight containers and away from excess heat and sunlight. I prefer to store my herbs in large mason jars with a tight-fitting lid and then placed them in a cupboard. If you have open shelves in your kitchen that do not receive direct sunlight then your jars of herbs would be a beautiful addition to your décor.

Herbs should maintain their potency in your mason jars for up to two years as long as they were dried properly. It would be wise to check them periodically to be certain there is no mold growth; A few ways to determine if your herbs are still good is to observe any changes in their color and aroma. If you find that they just don't look or smell right, then it is time to toss them.

6 Tips For Storing Dried Herbs

When putting together an herbal apothecary, dried herbs take center stage. Dried herbs are the first ingredient in so many different herbal preparations like herbal teas, infused oils, and tinctures. As one starts amassing a collection of dried herbs, it becomes increasingly important to be sure that you are storing dried herbs properly to ensure the highest level of potency.

The main culprits to the degradation of dried herbs are moisture, oxygen, sunlight, heat, and time. Different types of herbs also have different storage lives. Dried flowers and leaves will lose their potency faster than roots and seeds, for example. Keeping track of when the herbs were acquired is also important to have the highest quality herbs for your preparations. These 6 tips for storing dried herbs will greatly help you to increase their shelf life, keeping them fresh for as long as possible.

1. Whole Herbs Last Longer

The first thing to consider is that herbs in their whole form last longer. If you can store the whole herb and then grind them as needed, you will get a much fresher and stronger product. A good rule of thumb is to store them in the largest form that you can. Of course, this isn't always possible, and some herbs are easier to store in the whole form than others, such as roots, seeds, or whole flower buds.

2. Make Sure Your Herbs Are Dry

When you are preparing to store dried herbs, it's important to make sure that they are totally dry first. This applies if you are wildcrafting or harvesting fresh herbs from your backyard and then drying them for later use. You will want to make sure that there is absolutely no moisture left when they are finished drying. A good way to check is to rub a bit between your fingers—it should crumble easily and be almost crispy to the touch. A great way to dry your herbs is with a homemade drying screen, in a dehydrator, or by simply hanging them upside down.

3. Store In Airtight Containers

Oxygen will degrade herbs over time, so storing your dried herbs in airtight containers is best. Glass jars or metal tins with screw top lids work well, as do jars with clamp-on lips (Fido style). Avoid using plastic if possible, as it may leach chemicals into your herbs.

4. Keep Out Of Direct Sunlight

While those rays of sunlight hitting your jars of herbs might look pretty, they are doing damage to the potency of the herbs. For this reason, it's best to store them out of direct sunlight. Using dark-colored glass jars is even better for blocking all potential light. Keep them in a closed cabinet or make a curtain to cover them if need be.

5. Keep In A Cool And Dry Location

You want your herbs to stay cool and dry for maximum shelf life. Do not store them near a hot stove or in a steamy bathroom. A root cellar is ideal if you have one, or in a bedroom that is on the coolest side of your house.

6. Be Sure To Label Harvest Or Purchase Date

Keeping track of how old your herbs are is an important habit to develop. Whenever you put a new herb on the shelf, label what it is and when it was harvested or purchased.

Here Is A Good List To Follow When Labeling:

- ❖ Name
- ❖ Botanical name

- ❖ Harvest date (if known)
- ❖ Purchase date (if applicable)
- ❖ Discard date

Having the highest quality herbs is something that all herbalists should strive for, and it isn't hard if a little care is taken. Besides knowing that it's what is best for your herbs, it's also a good feeling to have a clean and organized apothecary. Labels with names and dates take all guesswork out of it, and you can get into a system of replenishing when the need arises. Make your herbal apothecary your space, treat it like a special place, and your dried herbs will last for quite a while. If you follow these 6 tips for storing dried herbs, you will have the freshest herbs possible in your herbal apothecary!

Herbal Preparation Methods

Infusion

This is often referred to as a "tea". An infusion is used to draw out the most fragile of healing properties of plants. Water is used to extract vitamins, some volatile oils, sugars, enzymes and other proteins, tannins, saponins, glycosides, bitter compounds, polysaccharides (when hot water used), pectins, and some alkaloids. Infusions are most often used with the softer parts of a plant – leaves, and flowers. There are a few exceptions, like Goldenseal root and Valerian root.

Infusions Can Be Done Hot Or Cold.

For a cold infusion, place the plant material in the cold water (I prefer steam distilled water) and allow it to "steep" for 4 to 8 hours, depending on the herb. This can be done at room temperature or in the fridge.

For a hot infusion, place 1 tsp. of the dried herb, or 2 tbsp. of the fresh herb in a cup pour 1 cup of boiling water over the herb cover and allow to steep for 10 minutes, or until cool enough to drink. These are very general guidelines and can be adjusted according to need or taste. If you are going to make a pint of infusion, adjust the amount of herb. If you need a stronger infusion, use more herbs.

Somewhere between the two is "sun tea" prepare the herbs as you would for a hot infusion, but pour room temperature water in the container. Tightly cover the container (a mason jar is great for this) and leave on a sunny window sill or outside in the sun for 4 to 8 hours. This works well. Herb "teas" can be soothing, refreshing, invigorating, and very healthful. They are the easiest of preparations and are quickly absorbed into your system.

Decoction

A decoction is used most often with more woody, resinous material, like roots, bark, seeds, and nuts. To make a decoction, use approximately the same amount of herb to water as for an infusion. You can either place the herbs in boiling water (at a very low boil, or simmer) or put the herbs in cold water and bring it up to a boil over low heat. The pot (NEVER use aluminum!) should have a tight-fitting lid. Once the water is simmering, cover and allow to simmer for approximately 20 minutes (some herbs need longer). Take off the heat, allow to cool, strain, and drink. Or, you can allow the decoction to steep all night, strain, and drink in the morning.

Juice

Some plants are best used for juicing the fresh plant. Fresh, spring picked nettles or wheatgrass is very nutritious this way. If you have a wheatgrass juicer, it can be used with other herbs. A Champion Juicer can be used if you combine the herb with some vegetables, like celery or carrot. Or, you can put the plant material in a blender with some pineapple juice, but some oxidation happens with this method, and you need to strain the liquid before drinking. If you happen to have a hydraulic press, you can also try pressing the plants to get the juice.

Fomentation

A fomentation is taking an infusion or decoction (often double or quadruple strength) and dipping some natural material (cotton, wool, silk) in the liquid, wringing out the excess liquid, and placing the soaked cloth over the affected area. You can also place a dry towel or cloth over the fomentation to keep it warm as long as possible, and some plastic wrap over that helps keep the liquid from dripping out.

Poultice

A poultice is the plant material itself placed over an affected area. Usually, the herb is bruised or macerated and placed over the injury or affected area, and covered with a bandage. It can be as simple as tearing up and bruising some yarrow leaves, and placing them over a cut, or putting some plantain leaves in your mouth, chewing them until they are a soft mass, and placing that over a bee sting. You can also use something like flaxseed to hold the herb in place. Grind up some flaxseed, mix in some of the powdered, fresh, or tinctured herb, and apply to the problem area. The ground flaxseed makes a sticky mass and may need nothing to hold it in place. If the flax seeds have been warmed up, this can be a warm poultice.

Oils

Extra virgin, cold-pressed olive oil is my oil of choice for making herbal oils. Olive oil takes a long time to go rancid at room temperature, and it is very nutritive in its own right. You can also use cold-pressed almond oil, grape seed oil, or apricot oil. These are especially good for facial products (considered cosmetic grade oils). Be sure to use the freshest, highest grade of oil.

You can use dried herbs or fresh herbs in your oil. If you use fresh herbs, make sure there is no excess moisture on the plant material. You can "wilt" the plants (let them dry in a warm place out of direct sunlight) for a few hours to be sure that there is no excess moisture.

Place your herbs in the container either a mason jar or a non-aluminum pan with a tight lid. Pour enough oil to cover the herbs and, in a mason jar, add 2 to 3 inches more of oil, or, in a non-aluminum pot, add another inch of oil. This keeps the herbs from poking out of the oil and attracting bacteria, which would spoil the oil.

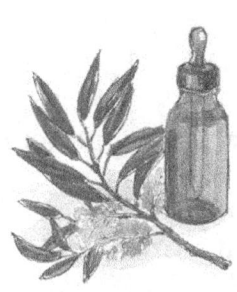

If you wish to infuse the oil, place a tight lid (for dried herbs) or a clean cloth held on with a rubber band (for fresh herbs) on the jar and put the jar in a sunny window for two weeks.

You can place your mason jar of herbs and oil in the oven as is, or in a pan of water so that the water comes halfway up the side of the jar in the oven. Turn the oven onto the lowest heat setting, and leave the jar in there for 1 to 3 hours. The temperature of the oil should never go above 120 degrees Fahrenheit.

For a faster oil, place the dried, fresh herbs in the top of a double boiler (glass or stainless steel) and cover with oil as instructed above. Cover, and bring the water up to a slow simmer. Keep it there for 30 minutes to 3 hours, depending on how hot the oil gets. As warned above, the oil should never get over

120 degrees Fahrenheit. Around 100 degrees is preferable. Keeping the oil at a lower temperature, longer, gives a better quality of the oil. Cool the oil and strain.

Store this in a dark bottle in a cool place.

Ointment / Salve

Once you've made the oil as above, making the ointment is fairly easy. For every cup of herbal oil, use 1/4 cup of grated beeswax. Bring your oil back up to temperature (not over 120 degrees) over a double boiler. I like to meet the bee's wax separately because it melts at a higher temperature. Melt the beeswax, and slowly pour it into your heated herbal oil, while stirring. Keep stirring until the liquid is consistent color, and is clear. To test the consistency, put a spoonful of the mixture in the freezer for a few minutes. If it is the hardness you want, then finish the preparation. If it is too soft, add a little more melted beeswax. If it is a little too hard, add a little more heated herbal oil.

Before cooling the mixture, you may add 8 drops of tincture of Benzoin for every cup of herbal oil you used, as a natural preservative. Take the mixture off the double boiler to cool. Add a few drops (don't go overboard!) of essential oil for a more pleasant aroma. Keep stirring the mixture until it just starts getting cloudy. This means it is ready to set up. Pour into small glass jars and seal. These can be kept in a cool, dark place, or even in the fridge. They should last for several months. If you start to see signs of spoilage or mold, throw them out.

Tincture / Liniment

Tinctures are an infusion in a menstruum of alcohol, vinegar, or glycerin. There are almost as many ways to make tinctures as there are herbalists. Most alcohol tinctures are made with grain alcohol – 80 to 100 proof vodka (this is 40 to 50% alcohol). You can use other things like wine, brandy, etc. to add a different flavor, but those have other ingredients in them. For some herbs, stronger alcohol needs to be used – in the range of 60 to 90% alcohol. You can adjust the alcohol level by adding some distilled water to the mix if you don't want 90% alcohol.

I fill a mason jar 1/2 to 3/4 full with dried or fresh herb material. Then I fill the jar to the top with the alcohol. I put a tight lid on the jar and shake it well. Leave this in a dark place for a minimum of 2 weeks shaking the bottle at least once a day, and preferably 3 times a day or more. Some herbalists leave the tinctures for up to 6 weeks. Some start the tinctures at the dark phase of the moon and strain it at the full moon. Try it in different ways.

When you are ready, strain the herbs through several layers of clean, cotton cloth or cheesecloth – I like to use flour sackcloth. Strain it several times, if need be, so there is no sediment. You want a clean tincture, so no bacteria will grow in it.

Pour the strained tincture into dark bottles and cap tightly. Keep them in a cool, dark place, and they should last for years.

Dosages of tinctures vary greatly depending on what herbs are used, on the age of the person, and if the health complaint is chronic or acute. It can be anywhere from 15 – 30 drops 3 times a day, to a teaspoon or more every hour. Tinctures can be taken straight. The healing properties will begin being absorbed into the system through the blood vessels in the mouth, especially if you drop the tincture under the tongue. Some people don't wish to take the alcohol or give it to children, so the tincture can be put into a cup of boiled water. Let it sit until the liquid is cool enough to drink, and most of the alcohol will have dissipated.

A vinegar tincture is made the same way using raw, apple cider vinegar. Use the same proportions of herbs to vinegar as in the alcohol tincture, and allow to infuse for 2 to 6 weeks. This makes a good tonic remedy, but it won't be as strong as an alcohol tincture. And you should start checking to see if it is still good after 6 to 8 months. A lot depends on where it is stored.

A glycerin tincture (a glycerite) is made the same way, using equal parts of pure vegetable glycerin to water, or using 2 parts glycerin to one part water. Make it the same as the alcohol tincture. This will draw out some healing properties from the herbs, but not as much as the alcohol. This is often used for children's formulas because glycerin is sweet.

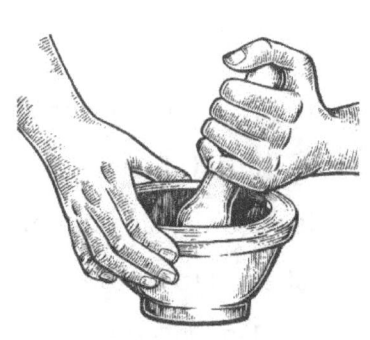

Now, liniments are essentially the same as a tincture but can be made with either rubbing alcohol (PLEASE be sure to mark the bottle for external use only!!!) or vinegar. Liniments are used as antiseptics on minor scrapes and wounds, or as a rub for sour muscles and joints.

Macerations

This method of preparation is certainly the easiest. The fresh or dried plant material is simply covered in cool water and soaked overnight. The herb is strained out and the liquid is taken. Normally this is used for very tender plants and/or fresh plants, or those with delicate chemicals that might be harmed by heating or which might be degraded in strong alcohol. This is also the easiest to adapt to western methods since tablets or capsules can be used instead. Alternatively, just stir the ground plant powder into juice, water, or smoothies and drink.

Syrup

This is a great way to prepare a formula for a child to take – or, for an adult, if the herbs are particularly bad tasting! I have seen several different ways of making syrups. Most of the old recipes use sugar… lots of it.

Start with 2 oz. of dried herb mix to 1 quart of water in a double boiler. Simmer this until you have 1 pint of liquid. Strain and pour the liquid back into the double boiler. For each pint of liquid, add a cup of raw honey. Heat this just enough so that the honey is mixed in with the herb decoction. Don't "cook" the honey.

When this is ready, take it off the heat to cool. Now, you can add a little fruit brandy (3 to 4 tbsp. per cup of syrup), or a few drops of essential oil, or a fruit concentrate for flavoring. The brandy is relaxing to the throat muscles, but if you are concerned about giving alcohol to children, then go with the essential oil or fruit concentrate. Peppermint, spearmint, or wintergreen essential oils are great.

Pour this into dark bottles, and keep it in the refrigerator. They will keep for several weeks to several months.

Powder / Capsules

This is an easy one... you can buy most herbs already powdered. Or, you can powder them, yourself, using a small coffee grinder (don't use one that has been used to grind the coffee, however!). If you grind your herbs, be sure to sift them to get any larger pieces out before encapsulating them. You can take the powdered herbs straight, swallowing it down with some herbal tea. However, I don't know of too many herbs that taste good enough for me to want to do this. I like to use the Capsule Machine for making my capsules.

Now, you can use the gelatin capsules, or, if you are vegetarian, you can get plant-based capsules. Why take capsules? Well, it takes longer for the herbs to get into your system with capsules, but you aren't losing any of the herbs, either. If you want to use the whole plant, capsules are the way to go. Take the capsules with warm, herbal tea. (Be careful with cayenne capsules, however – they can start to disintegrate in the throat, and you will feel the heat!)

Pills / Lozenge / Suppository

These are all made in similar ways – powdered herbs are added to a liquid until a stiff dough is formed. Then the mixture is shaped as needed.

For pills or lozenges, powdered herbs (usually for the throat or for a cough) are mixed with water and honey to make a paste. To this, add a few drops of essential oil, like peppermint or wintergreen. Thicken the mixture with enough Slippery elm, comfrey root, or marshmallow root powder to make the mixture's consistency like dough. Pinch off enough to make a small pill or a larger lozenge. Roll it into a ball and press between your fingers to flatten (they dry through faster in this shape, but you can leave them as balls). Then cover it with a little more Slippery elm powder or some carob powder. Place these pills/lozenges in a very low oven, in a dryer set on low, or in the sun for a day. Once they are dry, they will keep for a long time.

A suppository is similar, but the powdered herbs are mixed into melted cocoa butter. Cocoa butter is a hard fat at room temperature, but it melts at body temperature. This is a very good way to get herbs directly into the vagina, the rectum, or even in the nasal passages. Use about 1/2 oz. of powdered herbs to 3/4 to 1 oz. of melted cocoa butter. Stir until the mixture starts to thicken. Form the mixture into small cylinders, about 1/4" by 1" for the rectum or vagina. Put these on a plate and cover with a paper towel. When they are hardened, they can be used. Usually, the suppository is placed in the vaginal or rectal area just before going to bed, and it is wise to wear a pad in case any of the melted cocoa butter runs out.

For the nasal passages, form them into 1/8" by 1/4 to 1/2" cylinders. Harden them the same way. Place the suppository up into the nose. Prepare for running and sneezing as the cocoa butter melts and the herbs start to work.

Importance of Medicinal Plants And Herbs

Medicinal plants are considered as rich resources of ingredients that can be used in drug development either pharmacopoeial, non- pharmacopoeial, or synthetic drugs. Apart from that, these plants play a critical role in the development of human cultures around the whole world. Moreover, some plants are considered an important source of nutrition, and as a result that they are recommended for their therapeutic values. Some of these plants include ginger, green tea, walnuts, aloe, pepper, and turmeric, etc. Some plants and their derivatives are considered as an important source for active ingredients which are used in aspirin and toothpaste etc.

Apart from the medicinal uses, herbs are also used in natural dye, pest control, food, perfume, tea, and so on. In many countries, different kinds of medicinal plants/ herbs are used to keep ants, flies, mice, and flee away from homes and offices. Nowadays medicinal herbs are important sources for pharmaceutical manufacturing.

Recipes for the treatment of common ailments such as diarrhea, constipation, hypertension, low sperm count, dysentery and weak penile erection, piles, coated tongue, menstrual disorders, bronchial asthma, leucorrhoea, and fevers are given by the traditional medicine practitioners very effectively.

Importance of Some Herbs With Their Medicinal Values

1. Herbs such as black pepper, cinnamon, myrrh, aloe, sandalwood, ginseng, red clover, burdock, bayberry, and safflower are used to heal wounds, sores, and boils.

2. Basil, Fennel, Chives, Cilantro, Apple Mint, Thyme, Golden Oregano, Variegated Lemon Balm, Rosemary, Variegated Sage are some important medicinal herbs and can be planted in the kitchen garden. These herbs are easy to grow, look good, taste and smell amazing and many of them are magnets for bees and butterflies.

3. Many herbs are used as blood purifiers to alter or change a long-standing condition by eliminating the metabolic toxins. These are also known as 'blood cleansers'. Certain herbs improve the immunity of the person, thereby reducing conditions such as fever.

4. Some herbs are also having antibiotic properties. Turmeric is useful in inhibiting the growth of germs, harmful microbes, and

bacteria. Turmeric is widely used as a home remedy to heal cuts and wounds.

5. Sandalwood and Cinnamon are great astringents apart from being aromatic. Sandalwood is especially used in arresting the discharge of blood, mucus, etc.

6. Some herbs are used to neutralize the acid produced by the stomach. Herbs such as marshmallow root and leaf. They serve as antacids. The healthy gastric acid needed for proper digestion is retained by such herbs.

7. Herbs like Cardamom and Coriander are renowned for their appetizing qualities. Other aromatic herbs such as peppermint, cloves, and turmeric add a pleasant aroma to the food, thereby increasing the taste of the meal.

8. Some herbs like aloe, sandalwood, and turmeric are commonly used as antiseptic and are very high in their medicinal values.

9. Ginger and cloves are used in certain cough syrups. They are known for their expectorant property, which promotes the thinning and ejection of mucus from the lungs, trachea, and bronchi. Eucalyptus, Cardamom, Wild cherry, and cloves are also expectorants.

10. Herbs such as Chamomile, Calamus, Ajwain, Basil, Cardamom, Chrysanthemum, Coriander, Fennel, Peppermint,

and Spearmint, Cinnamon, Ginger, and Turmeric help promote good blood circulation. Therefore, they are used as cardiac stimulants.

11. Certain medicinal herbs have disinfectant property, which destroys disease-causing germs. They also inhibit the growth of pathogenic microbes that cause communicable diseases.

12. Certain aromatic plants such as Aloe, Goldenseal, Barberry, and Chirayata are used as mild tonics. The bitter taste of such plants reduces toxins in the blood. They help destroy infection as well.

13. A wide variety of herbs including Giloe, Goldenseal, Aloe, and Barberry are used as tonics. They can also be nutritive and rejuvenate a healthy as well as the diseased individual.

14. Honey, turmeric, marshmallow, and licorice can effectively treat a fresh cut and wound. They are termed as vulnerable herbs.

Misuse of Medicinal Plants And Herbs

Misuse refers to patient overdosing and concomitant drug consumption. Kava, for example, is used as an anxiolytic and a mild tranquilizer in dosing ranging from 60 to 120mg of kava pyrones daily. Some users may consume as much as triple this amount for extended periods without concern for the potentially dangerous effects, which include malnutrition, liver, and renal dysfunction, and pulmonary hypertension.

Some Other Common Misuses Of Medicinal Herbs/Products

- ❖ Carelessness with prescriptions and medical drugs
- ❖ Nonprofessionals making prescriptions and selling, unaware of harmful side effects
- ❖ Uneducated people using medicinal plants.
- ❖ Alternative medicine- a common misconception is that they are safer than man-made drugs because they are natural.
- ❖ Only certified doctors and professionals have regulated the strength and dosage of the medicinal ingredients.

Tips For Using Medicinal Herbs Safely

- ❖ Buy or use herbal products from a qualified practitioner or reputable supplier.
- ❖ Ask for products that are clearly labeled in English with your name, batch number, date, quantity, dosage, directions, safety information (if applicable), and your practitioner's contact details.
- ❖ Avoid using over-the-counter products from a health food shop, pharmacy, or the internet.
- ❖ Make sure you know how to prepare and take your herbs. Like conventional medicine, taking the correct dose at

the right time is important for herbal remedies to work safely.
- ❖ Talk to your doctor and complementary health practitioner
- ❖ Ask the practitioner for ways to mask the taste of the herbs if you find them bitter.

Essential Tools And Useful Instruments

1. Felco Pruners

Pruners are the tool I use most often when gathering and processing foraged herbs. They snip right through herbaceous stems, twigs, small branches, and roots. I reach for them so often that I keep them in a leather holster on a belt at my hip. If you can only purchase one tool to get started, pruners are the way to go!. Felco pruners come in a wide variety of models. Look for a pair that will reduce hand fatigue and strain. The pruner handles, when fully opened, should not exceed the width of your extended grasp.

2. Hori-Hori, Or Weeding Knife, Or Japanese Garden Knife

This tool looks like it sounds. Heavy duty and compact, it's a sturdy wildcrafting tool and excellent weeding implement. I use my hori-hori to break up soils and dig small- to medium-sized roots from the earth. These garden "knives" cut through most clay soils and can even pry rocks out of the ground. You can also use it for transplanting and dividing roots.

3. Digging Fork

This is the tool of choice for digging most roots. The tines of the fork effectively loosen soils and lift branching roots free from the earth. Digging forks are much less likely to damage roots than a shovel or spade. I also use my digging fork in the garden to weed, loosen soil, and harvest medicinal roots.

4. Shovel

You likely already have this tool hanging out in your garage or garden shed. Having a couple of different types is useful. Make sure you have at least one long-handled shovel with a pointed blade (as opposed to flat). It is used primarily to help begin the excavation process of large, tap-rooted plants like burdock (Arctium lappa, A. minus), or digging in heavily compacted soils.

5. Kitchen Scissors

A sharp pair of kitchen scissors is my go-to tool for gathering tender-stemmed greens like chickweed (Stellaria media), violet (Viola spp.), and cleavers (Galium aparine). Pruners can make a muck of this job as they're meant for tougher stems and the reach of their blades is limited.

6. Pruning Saw

A foldable pruning saw is handy for cutting small- to medium-sized tree limbs and branches. I use mine most often in the spring when I'm gathering medicinal tree barks like wild cherry (Prunus serotina) and black birch (Betula lenta).

7. Assorted Baskets

Baskets will reward you in more ways than one. They're handy for gathering and drying herbs, and they are beautiful to behold. It's helpful to have an assortment of baskets on hand. You can typically find used baskets in thrift stores. Look for a few that have an open weave and are broad and flattish (helpful for increasing ventilation when drying loose herbs).

9. Gloves

Foraging can be hard on the hands, and your fingertips will thank you for stashing a pair of gloves in your pack for prickly situations (think: picking stinging nettles or wading through a berry bramble). I keep two pairs of gloves on hand a thin, supple pair for delicate tasks and thicker leather and/or canvas pair for moments when I need more protection.

10. Hand Lens Or Loupe

I highly recommend purchasing a hand lens, also called a jeweler's loupe preferably 10x to 20x (10 to 20 times magnification). These nifty little tools allow you to gaze at wee botanical parts (helpful for plant ID) and have a much higher magnification ability than plain magnifying lenses (the kind used for enlarging print). Many have an LED attached, which is ideal because the increased lighting makes it much easier to spy on flowers.

CHAPTER 3 : NATIVE AMERICAN HERBS

1. Aloe - Aloe Doctrina

Aloe is a cactus-like plant that grows in hot, dry climates. In the United States, aloe is grown in Florida, Texas, and Arizona. Aloe produces two substances, gel, and latex, which are used for medicines. Aloe gel is the clear, jelly-like substance found in the inner part of the aloe plant leaf. Aloe latex comes from just under the plant's skin and is yellow. Some aloe products are made from the whole crushed leaf, so they contain both gel and latex. The aloe that is mentioned in the Bible is an unrelated fragrant wood used as incense.

Aloe medications can be taken by mouth or applied to the skin. People take aloe products by mouth for conditions such as obesity, diabetes, osteoarthritis, and many others, but there is no good scientific evidence to support these uses. People apply aloe gel to the skin for conditions such as acne, dandruff, wound healing, and many others, but there is no good scientific evidence to support these uses.

How Does It Work?

The useful parts of aloe are the gel and latex. The gel is obtained from the cells in the center of the leaf, and the latex is obtained from the cells just beneath the leaf skin. Aloe gel might cause changes in the skin that might help diseases like psoriasis. Aloe seems to be able to speed wound healing by improving blood circulation through the area and preventing cell death around a wound. It also appears that aloe gel has properties that are harmful to certain types of bacteria and fungi. Aloe latex contains chemicals that work as a laxative.

Uses & Effectiveness

Possibly Effective For

- Acne.
- Burns
- Constipation.
- Diabetes.
- Genital herpes.
- Scaly, itchy skin (psoriasis).
- Possibly Ineffective for
- Burning pain in the mouth.
- HIV/AIDS.

Special Precautions & Warnings:

1. Pregnancy Or Breast-Feeding: Aloe either gel or latex is POSSIBLY UNSAFE when taken by mouth. There is a report that aloe was associated with miscarriage. It might also increase the risk of birth defects. Do not take aloe by mouth if you are pregnant or breast-feeding.

2. Children: Aloe gel is POSSIBLY SAFE when applied to the skin appropriately. Aloe latex and aloe whole leaf extracts are POSSIBLY UNSAFE when taken by mouth in children. Children younger than 12 years-old might have stomach pain, cramps, and diarrhea.

3. Diabetes: Some research suggests that aloe might lower blood sugar. If you take aloe by mouth and you have diabetes, monitor your blood sugar levels closely.

4. Hemorrhoids: Do not take aloe latex if you have hemorrhoids. It could make the condition worse. Remember, products made from whole aloe leaves will contain some aloe latex.

5. Kidney Problems: High doses of aloe latex have been linked to kidney failure and other serious conditions.

6. Surgery: Aloe might affect blood sugar levels and could interfere with blood sugar control during and after surgery. Stop taking aloe at least 2 weeks before a scheduled surgery.

Interactions

Major Interaction

- ❖ Do not take this combination
- ❖ Digoxin (Lanoxin) interacts with ALOE

When taken by mouth aloe latex is a type of laxative called a stimulant laxative. Stimulant laxatives can decrease potassium levels in the body. Low potassium levels can increase the risk of side effects of digoxin (Lanoxin).

Moderate Interaction

Be cautious with this combination

1. Medications Taken By Mouth (Oral Drugs) Interacts With ALOE

When taken by mouth aloe latex is a laxative. Laxatives can decrease how much medicine your body absorbs. Taking aloe latex along with medications you take by mouth might decrease the effectiveness of your medication.

2. Sevoflurane (Ultane) Interacts With ALOE

Aloe might decrease the clotting of the blood. Sevoflurane is used as anesthesia during surgery. Sevoflurane also decreases the clotting of the blood. Taking aloe before surgery might cause increased bleeding during the surgical procedure. Do not take aloe by mouth if you are having surgery within 2 weeks.

3. Stimulant Laxatives Interact With ALOE

When taken orally aloe latex is a type of laxative called a stimulant laxative. Stimulant laxatives speed up the bowels. Taking aloe latex along with other stimulant laxatives could speed up the bowels too much and cause dehydration and low minerals in the body.

4. Warfarin (Coumadin) Interacts With ALOE

When taken orally, aloe latex is a type of laxative called a stimulant laxative. Stimulant laxatives speed up the bowels and can cause diarrhea in some people. Diarrhea can increase the effects of warfarin and increase the risk of bleeding. If you take warfarin, do not take excessive amounts of aloe latex.

5. Water Pills (Diuretic Drugs) Interacts With ALOE

When taken by mouth aloe latex is a laxative. Some laxatives can decrease potassium in the body. "Water pills" can also decrease potassium in the body. Taking aloe latex along with "water pills" might decrease potassium in the body too much. Some "water pills" that can decrease potassium include chlorothiazide (Diuril), chlorthalidone (Thalitone), furosemide

(Lasix), hydrochlorothiazide (HCTZ, HydroDIURIL, Microzide), and others.

Dosing

The following doses have been studied in scientific research:

1. Adults

By Mouth:

1. For Constipation: 100-200 mg of aloe or 50 mg of aloe extract taken in the evening has been used. Also, a 500 mg capsule containing aloe, starting at a dose of one capsule daily and increasing to three capsules daily as required, has been used.

2. For Diabetes: The most effective dose and form of aloe for diabetes is unclear. Multiple doses and forms of aloe have been used for 4-14 weeks, including powder, extract, and juice. Doses of powder range from 100-1000 mg daily. Doses of juice range from 15-150 mL daily.

3. For Obesity: A specific aloe gel product containing 147 mg of aloe twice daily for 8 weeks has been used.

4. For A Painful Mouth Disease That Reduces One's Ability To Open The Mouth (Oral Submucous Fibrosis): Pure aloe vera juice 30 mL twice daily along with applying pure aloe vera gel to lesions three times daily for 3 months has been used.

Applied To The Skin:

1. For Acne: A 50% aloe gel has been applied in the morning and evening after washing the face, along with a prescription called tretinoin gel in the evening.

2. For Burns: Aloe and olive oil cream, applied twice daily for 6 weeks, has been used. Also, aloe gel or cream applied twice or three times daily after changing a wound dressing, or every three days until the burn heals, has been used.

3. For Genital Herpes: A cream containing 0.5% aloe extract, applied three times daily for 5 consecutive days once or twice over 2 weeks, has been used.

4. For An Inflammatory Condition That Causes Rash Or Sores On The Skin Or Mouth (Lichen Planus): Aloe gel, applied two to three times daily for 8 weeks has been used. Two tablespoons of aloe mouthwash swished for 2 minutes and then spit, four times daily for one month has been used.

5. For Scaly, Itchy Skin (Psoriasis): Aloe extract 0.5% cream applied three times daily for 4 weeks has been used. A cream containing aloe applied twice daily for 8 weeks, has been used.

Children

Applied To The Skin:

1. For Acne: A 50% aloe gel has been applied in the morning and evening after washing the face, along with a prescription called tretinoin gel in the evening.

2. For A Painful Mouth Disease That Reduces One's Ability To Open The Mouth (Oral Submucous Fibrosis): 5 mg of an aloe gel, applied on each side of the cheeks three times daily for 3 months, has been used.

2. Arsesmart - Polygonum Hydropiper

What Is Smartweed?

Smartweed is an herb. The entire plant is used to make medicine. People take smartweed tea to stop bleeding from hemorrhoids, as well as menstrual bleeding and another uterine bleeding. They also use it to treat diarrhea. Some people put smartweed directly on the skin to wash bloody wounds.

Insufficient Evidence To Rate Effectiveness For

- ❖ Stopping bleeding.
- ❖ Diarrhea.
- ❖ Cleansing bloody wounds, when applied directly.
- ❖ Other conditions.

How Does Smartweed Work?

Smartweed contains chemicals that are thought to stop bleeding.

Are There Safety Concerns?

It is not known if smartweed is safe. It can cause side effects such as stomach irritation when taken by mouth. When the fresh plant is handled it can cause skin irritation and swelling (inflammation).

Special Precautions & Warnings:

1. Pregnancy And Breast-Feeding: Not enough is known about the use of smartweed during pregnancy and breast-feeding. Stay on the safe side and avoid use.

Ulcers Or Other Stomach And Intestinal (Gastrointestinal, GI) Disorders: Smartweed can irritate the tissues that line the stomach and intestines, making ulcers and GI problems worse. Avoid using smartweed if you have ulcers or another GI disorder.

Are There Any Interactions With Medications?

Warfarin (Coumadin)Interaction Rating: Moderate Be cautious with this combination. Talk with your health provider.

Smartweed contains large amounts of vitamin K. Vitamin K is used by the body to help blood clot. Warfarin (Coumadin) is used to slow blood clotting. By helping the blood clot, smartweed might decrease the effectiveness of warfarin (Coumadin). Be sure to have your blood checked regularly. The dose of your warfarin (Coumadin) might need to be changed.

Dosing Considerations For Smartweed

The appropriate dose of smartweed depends on several factors such as the user's age, health, and several other conditions. At this time there is not enough scientific information to determine an appropriate range of doses for smartweed. Keep in mind that natural products are not always necessarily safe and dosages can be important. Be sure to follow relevant directions on product labels and consult your pharmacist or physician or other healthcare professional before using.

3. Black Cohosh - Cimicifuga Racemosa

Generic Name: Black Cohosh

Drug Class: Women's Health, Herbals

What Is Black Cohosh (Vasostrict, Adh) And How Does It Work?

Black Cohosh suggested uses include cough, sore throat, painful menstrual periods (dysmenorrhea), indigestion/heartburn, labor induction, menopausal symptoms, nervous tension, premenstrual syndrome, and rheumatism.

Black Cohosh is likely effective for menopausal vasomotor symptoms. Black Cohosh is possibly effective for premenstrual syndrome (PMS) and painful menstrual periods (dysmenorrhea). Black Cohosh is available under the following different brands and other names: Actaea racemosa, baneberry, black snakeroot, bugbane, bugwort, Cimicifuga racemosa, rattle root, rattlesnake root, rattleweed, rheumatism weed, and squawroot.

Dosages Of Black Cohosh:

Suggested Dosing

Dried Root: 300-2000 mg orally three times daily

Extract: 0.3-2 mL orally daily; 1:1, 90% alcohol

Tincture: 2-4 mL orally daily; 1:10, 60% alcohol

Tablet: 20-80 mg orally twice daily; standardized to 1 mg triterpene glycosides/20 mg tablet

What Are Side Effects Associated With Using Black Cohosh?

Side effects of Black Cohosh include:

- ❖ Cramping
- ❖ Dizziness
- ❖ Gastrointestinal (GI) upset
- ❖ Headache
- ❖ Sweating

- ❖ Weight gain
- ❖ Rash
- ❖ Fast heart rate (overdose)
- ❖ CNS disturbances
- ❖ Nausea
- ❖ Vomiting
- ❖ Visual disturbances

This document does not contain all possible side effects and others may occur. Check with your physician for additional information about side effects.

What Other Drugs Interact With Black Cohosh?

If your doctor has directed you to use this medication, your doctor or pharmacist may already be aware of any possible drug interactions and may be monitoring you for them. Do not start, stop, or change the dosage of any medicine before checking with your doctor, health care provider, or pharmacist first.

Black Cohosh has no known severe interactions with other drugs.

Serious interactions of black cohosh include:

- ❖ Daclizumab
- ❖ Black cohosh has no known moderate interactions with other drugs.

Mild interactions of black cohosh include:

- Nevirapine
- Tamoxifen
- Tenofovir df
- Zidovudine

This document does not contain all possible interactions. Therefore, before using this product, tell your doctor or pharmacist of all the products you use. Keep a list of all your medications with you, and share the list with your doctor and pharmacist. Check with your physician if you have health questions or concerns.

What Are Warnings And Precautions For Black Cohosh (Vasostrict, Adh)?

Warnings

This medication contains black cohosh. Do not take Actaea racemosa, baneberry, black snakeroot, bugbane, bugwort, Cimicifuga rattle root, rattlesnake root, rattleweed, rheumatism weed, or squawroot if you are allergic to black cohosh or any ingredients contained in this drug. Keep out of reach of children. In case of overdose, get medical help or contact a Poison Control Center immediately.

Contraindications

Breast cancer, endometrial cancer, endometriosis, hormone-sensitive conditions, ovarian cancer, pregnancy, lactation, uterine fibroids

Cautions

It May be associated with liver damage

Pregnancy And Lactation

Black cohosh is considered unsafe to use during pregnancy or while breastfeeding.

4. Black Root - Veronicastrum Virgin Icum

What Is Black Root?

Blackroot is a plant. It grows in the US and Canada and has a bitter and nauseating taste. People use the underground stem (rhizome) and the root as medicine. Blackroot is used for ongoing constipation and disorders of the liver and gallbladder. It is also used to cause vomiting.

Insufficient Evidence To Rate Effectiveness For

- ❖ Constipation.
- ❖ Liver problems.
- ❖ Gallbladder problems.
- ❖ Causing vomiting.

❖ Other conditions.

How Does Black Rootwork?

Blackroot might increase bile flow from the gallbladder into the intestine.

Are There Safety Concerns?

There isn't enough information to know if taking black root is safe. However, there have been reports of stomach pain or cramps, changes in stool color or odor, drowsiness, headache, nausea, and vomiting after taking black root. Large doses have been linked to reports of liver damage.

Special Precautions & Warnings:

1. Pregnancy And Breast-Feeding: It might be UNSAFE to take the fresh root by mouth. There is a concern that it might cause miscarriages and birth defects, but this hasn't been proven so far. Stay safe and don't take black root if you are pregnant. It's also best to avoid black roots if you are breast-feeding. Not enough is known about how it might affect the nursing infant.

2. Gallbladder Problems Such As Gallstones Or A Blocked Bile Duct: Don't take black root if you have gallbladder problems. It might make your condition worse.

3. Hemorrhoids: Don't use black roots if you have hemorrhoids. It can act as a laxative and make hemorrhoids more bothersome.

4. Menstruation: Don't take black root if you are having your period. It can act as a laxative and add to the discomfort.

Are There Any Interactions With Medications?

1. Digoxin (Lanoxin)Interaction Rating: Moderate Be cautious with this combination. Talk with your health provider.

2. Blackroot Is High In Fiber: Fiber can decrease the absorption and decrease the effectiveness of digoxin (Lanoxin). As a general rule, any medications taken by mouth should be taken one hour before or four hours after the black root to prevent this interaction.

3. Warfarin (Coumadin)Interaction Rating: Moderate Be cautious with this combination. Talk with your health provider.

4. Water Pills (Diuretic drugs)Interaction Rating: Moderate Be cautious with this combination. Talk with your health provider.

5. Blackroot Is A Laxative: Some laxatives can decrease potassium in the body. "Water pills" can also decrease potassium in the body. Taking black root along with "water pills" might decrease potassium in the body too much.

Dosing Considerations For Black Root

The appropriate dose of black root depends on several factors such as the user's age, health, and several other conditions. At this time there is not enough scientific information to determine an appropriate range of doses for black root. Keep in mind that natural products are not always necessarily safe and dosages can be important. Be sure to follow relevant directions on product labels and consult your pharmacist or physician or other healthcare professional before using.

5. Black Walnut - Juglans Nigra

What Are Black Walnuts?

Black walnuts, or Juglans nigra, grow wild across the United States and are the second most cultivated walnut in North America, following English walnuts. They consist of a kernel, a dry outer covering known as a hull, and a hard shell. The kernel is the part of the walnut that's commonly eaten raw or roasted and can be pressed for oil. The hulls contain antioxidants and are used in extracts and supplements for medicinal purposes, such as to treat parasitic infections or decrease inflammation. Black walnuts have a unique flavor and aroma, making them bolder and earthier than English walnuts. They're a popular addition to recipes like baked goods and desserts. Black walnuts are the second most common walnut and prized for their bold and earthy flavor. The nutrients in the hulls are extracted and used in supplements.

Black Walnut Nutrition

Black walnuts are high in protein, healthy fats, and many vitamins and minerals. A 1-ounce (28-gram) serving of black walnuts contains:

- Calories: 170
- Protein: 7 grams
- Fat: 17 grams
- Carbs: 3 grams
- Fiber: 2 grams
- Magnesium: 14% of the Reference Daily Intake (RDI)
- Phosphorus: 14% of the RDI
- Potassium: 4% of the RDI
- Iron: 5% of the RDI
- Zinc: 6% of the RDI
- Copper: 19% of the RDI
- Manganese: 55% of the RDI
- Selenium: 7% of the RDI

Potential Health Benefits Of Black Walnut

The fiber, omega-3 fatty acids, and antioxidants in black walnuts provide various health benefits. Also, black walnut hulls have unique antibacterial properties and are used in herbal medicine extracts and supplements. Black walnuts are nutritionally similar to English walnuts, which have been studied extensively for their health benefits.

May Benefit Heart Health

Black walnuts contain various nutrients and compounds that benefit heart health, including:

- Omega-3 fatty acids. May improve certain heart disease risk factors like high blood pressure and cholesterol levels.
- Tannins. Help lower blood pressure and decrease blood lipid levels, potentially improving heart health.
- Ellagic acid. May help prevent a narrowing of the arteries caused by plaque buildup that can lead to heart disease.

May Have Anticancer Properties

Black walnuts contain an antitumor compound called juglone. Test-tube studies have found this compound to significantly reduce tumor growth Several test-tube studies indicate that juglone can cause cell death in certain cancerous cells, including the liver and stomach Also, black walnuts contain flavonoid antioxidants that have been shown to have beneficial effects against lung, breast, prostate, and colon cancer.

Have Antibacterial Properties

Black walnut hulls are high in tannins compounds with antibacterial properties. Tannins in black walnuts have antibacterial effects against, for example, Listeria, Salmonella, and E. coli bacteria that commonly cause foodborne illnesses. A test-tube study found that black walnut hull extracts have antioxidant and antibacterial activities, preventing the growth of Staphylococcus aureus, a bacteria that can cause infections.

May Aid Weight Loss

Studies show that eating nuts particularly walnuts may help you lose weight Though walnuts are high in calories, most of these calories come from healthy fats. Fats can help increase feelings of fullness and fend off hunger. Walnuts have been found to keep you fuller for longer, which can help you naturally eat less, potentially promoting weight loss. In one 3-month study, people who ate 1/4 cup (30 grams) of walnuts daily experienced greater weight loss than the control group despite the additional calories of the walnuts

Black Walnut Uses

Plant compounds in black walnut hulls are extracted and used as supplements in the form of capsules or liquid drops. Due to its antibacterial properties, the black walnut extract is used in wormwood complex supplements. Wormwood complex is a tincture made from black walnut hulls, a plant called wormwood, and cloves. It's a natural remedy against parasitic infections.

Safety Of Black Walnut

Although black walnuts have many health benefits, there are some safety aspects to consider when eating them or taking them as a supplement. People with any nut or tree nut allergy should not eat black walnuts or use supplements that contain them. Supplements are not regulated by the Food and Drug Administration (FDA). Therefore, you should purchase them from reputable brands that offer products that are independently tested for safety and potency.

Research on the effects of black walnut supplements during pregnancy or while breastfeeding is insufficient, and it's unknown whether it's safe to take these supplements during pregnancy or lactation. Additionally, the tannins in black walnuts may interact with certain medications. It's best to consult with your healthcare provider before taking black walnut extract if you take medications or are pregnant or breastfeeding

6. Bloodroot - Sanguinaria Canadensis

Bloodroot is a plant. People use the underground stem (rhizome) to make medicine. People sometimes use bloodroot by mouth or apply it to the skin for a long list of conditions, but there is no scientific evidence to support these uses, and using it can be unsafe.

How Does It Work?

Bloodroot contains chemicals that might help fight bacteria, inflammation, and plaque.

Uses & Effectiveness?

Possibly Effective For

- ❖ Dental plaque.
- ❖ Swelling of the gums (gingivitis).
- ❖ Insufficient Evidence for
- ❖ Coughs.
- ❖ Spasms.
- ❖ Emptying the bowels.
- ❖ Causing vomiting.
- ❖ Wound cleaning.
- ❖ Other conditions.

Side Effects & Safety

Bloodroot is POSSIBLY SAFE for most people when taken by mouth, short-term. Side effects include nausea, vomiting, drowsiness, and grogginess.

Long-term use by mouth in high amounts is POSSIBLY UNSAFE. At high doses, it can cause low blood pressure, shock, coma, and an eye disease called glaucoma. Also, bloodroot is

POSSIBLY UNSAFE when used as a toothpaste, mouthwash, or applied to the skin. Don't let bloodroot get into your eyes because it can irritate. It may also cause white patches on the inside of the mouth. Skin contact with the fresh plant can cause a rash. Bloodroot can also burn and erode the skin, leaving an uneven scar.

Special Precautions & Warnings:

1. Pregnancy And Breast-Feeding: Bloodroot is LIKELY UNSAFE when taken by mouth during pregnancy and POSSIBLY UNSAFE when taken by mouth while breast-feeding; avoid use.

2. An Eye Disease Called Glaucoma: Bloodroot might affect glaucoma treatment. If you have glaucoma, don't use bloodroot unless a healthcare professional recommends it and monitors your eye health.

Dosing

The appropriate dose of bloodroot depends on several factors such as the user's age, health, and several other conditions. At this time there is not enough scientific information to determine an appropriate range of doses for bloodroot. Keep in mind that natural products are not always necessarily safe and dosages can be important. Be sure to follow relevant directions on product labels and consult your pharmacist or physician or other healthcare professional before using.

7. Bearberry - Uva Urst

Uva ursi is a shrub that grows flowers and berries. The leaves are used to make medicine. Bears are particularly fond of uva ursi berries. This explains the Latin name, "uva ursi," which means "bear's grape." Most authorities refer to Arctostaphylos uva-ursi as uva ursi. Do not confuse this plant with Arctostaphylos adentricha and Arctostaphylos coactylis, which have also been referred to as uva ursi. Uva ursi is used for infections of the kidney, bladder, or urethra (urinary tract infections or UTIs) and swelling (inflammation) of the urinary tract, but there is no good scientific evidence to support these uses.

How Does It Work?

Uva ursi can reduce bacteria in the urine. It can also reduce swelling (inflammation), and have a drying (astringent) effect on the tissues.

Uses & Effectiveness?

Insufficient Evidence For

- ❖ Swelling of the bladder and urethra.

- ❖ Swelling of the urinary tract.
- ❖ Constipation.
- ❖ Kidney infections.
- ❖ Bronchitis.
- ❖ Other conditions.

Side Effects & Safety

When taken by mouth: Uva ursi is POSSIBLY SAFE for most adults when taken for up to one month. It can cause nausea, vomiting, stomach discomfort, and a greenish-brown discoloration of the urine. But uva ursi is POSSIBLY UNSAFE when taken in high doses for more than one month. It can cause liver damage, breathing problems, convulsions, and death when used in high doses. When used for a long time, it might increase the risk of cancer.

Special Precautions & Warnings:

1. Pregnancy And Breast-Feeding: Using uva ursi during pregnancy is LIKELY UNSAFE because it might start labor. There isn't enough reliable information to know if uva ursi is safe to use when breastfeeding. Stay on the safe side and avoid use.

2. Children: Uva ursi is POSSIBLY UNSAFE in children when taken bymouth. Uva ursi contains a chemical that might cause severe liver problems. Do not give uva ursi to children.

3. Retinal Thinning: Uva ursi contains a chemical that can thin the retina in the eye. This could worsen the condition of people whose retinas are already too thin. Avoid use if you have this problem.

Dosing

The appropriate dose of uva ursi depends on several factors such as the user's age, health, and several other conditions. At this time there is not enough scientific information to determine an appropriate range of doses for uva ursi. Keep in mind that natural products are not always necessarily safe and dosages can be important. Be sure to follow relevant directions on product labels and consult your pharmacist or physician or other healthcare professional before using.

8. Capsicum - Capsicum Minimum, C. Frutescens

Capsicum

Capsicums, available in a multitude of colors, is an excellent source of vitamins A and C. This versatile vegetable can be stuffed, roasted, used in stir-fries, or simply eaten raw. In Victoria, capsicums are at their peak between March and November.

Also Called: peppers, sweet peppers, red pepper, green pepper, red capsicum, green capsicum, bell pepper, red bell pepper, green bell pepper, banana capsicum, Capsicum annuum L. (botanical name)

What Is Capsicum?

The rainbow of colors in which capsicum appears in Australia hints at the versatility of this vegetable – stuff it with herbs, meat, and rice, roast and use the smoky flesh in dips or simply eat it raw as a crudité, a traditional French appetizer. First prepared by herdsman as a hearty meal, the delicious Hungarian goulash wouldn't be the same without the addition of capsicum. The Capsicum species originated in South and Central America, and Christopher Columbus brought it back to Europe when he returned from the Americas. Records show that capsicum has been used in cooking since 6000 BC. In Australia, capsicum became popular thanks to European and Asian immigrants who use it extensively.

Why Capsicum Is Good To Eat

- ❖ Capsicums are an excellent source of vitamin A and C (red contain more than green capsicums).
- ❖ They are also a good source of dietary fiber, vitamin E, B6, and folate.
- ❖ The sweetness of capsicums is due to their natural sugars (green capsicums have less sugar than red capsicums).
- ❖ Energy 100 g of green capsicum supplies 90 kJ (105 kJ from red capsicum).

How Are They Grown And Harvested?

- ❖ Capsicums grow on a flowering bush that can reach up to 60 or 80 cm. Capsicum plants prefer stable, warm climates and are usually planted as seedlings.
- ❖ The seedlings take from 11 to 13 weeks to grow into mature plants with the capsicums ready to harvest. Red capsicums start green but if left on the bush to ripen they eventually turn red. Other types of capsicum turn yellow, orange, brown, or purple/black.
- ❖ Take care when you harvest capsicums. Rough treatment can injure the plant as the stems are very brittle and can snap off easily.

Choosing Capsicum

When choosing capsicums you should select ones with the firm, glossy skins. Avoid those with shriveled skins, soft spots, or other visible damage.

How To Store And Keep Capsicum

Store capsicums in the crisper section of your fridge. Ordinary plastic bags cause capsicums to sweat, so only use fridge storage bags. Capsicum should be used within five days.

How To Use

- To help remove the blackened skin of roasted peppers, place them in a plastic bag and allow them to cool for 10 minutes.
- For a Mediterranean flavor remove the stem and stuff red and green capsicums with a mixture of rice, tomato, pine nuts, and fresh herbs and bake until soft and tender.
- For a fresh, tangy salsa to accompany grilled fish mix chopped roasted red and yellow peppers, a small chili, coriander leaf, red onion, and dress with red wine vinegar oil and lime.
- Make a delicious savory dip by pureeing roasted peppers, garlic, capers, and fresh herbs with oil and lemon juice.

9. Catnip - Nepeta Cataria

Catnip, (Nepeta cataria), also called catmint, herb of the mint family (Lamiaceae), noted for its aromatic leaves, which are particularly exciting to cats. Catnip is commonly grown by cat owners for their pets, and the dried leaves are often used as a stuffing for cat playthings. The herb is native to Eurasia and is used as a seasoning and as a medicinal tea for colds and fever in some places. Catnip (nepeta cataria) is a fun plant for cats. Most cats are attracted to the plant and will roll around near it since its aroma acts as a stimulant. These medicinal plants also act as a sedative for cats if consumed.

For humans, on the other hand, it is normally used as a stress reliever, sleep aid, and a solution for skin issues. The majority of its health benefits come from the presence of nepetalactone, thymol, and other compounds that make this plant great for you and your furry friend.

Catnip Health Benefits:

- Repels bugs and relieves irritation from bug bites
- Calms restlessness, anxiety, and stress
- Relieves stomach discomfort
- Accelerates recovery from colds and fevers

Common uses:

- Brew leaves for a tea
- Dry leaves and burn to release the aroma
- Apply essential oils or leaves topically

10. Chamomile - Chamaemelum Nobile

Chamaemelum Nobile has daisy-like white flowers and procumbent stems; the leaves are alternate, bipinnate, finely dissected, and downy to glabrous. The solitary, terminal flowerheads, rising 20–30 cm (8–12 in) above the ground, consist of prominent yellow disk flowers and silver-white ray flowers. The flowering time in the Northern Hemisphere is June and July, and its fragrance is sweet, crisp, fruity, and herbaceous. Although the plant is often confused with German chamomile (M. chamomilla), its morphology, properties, and chemical composition are markedly different

Uses

- Chamaemelum Nobile has been used traditionally in hair care and skin care products. The plant may be used to flavor foods, in herbal teas, perfumes, and cosmetics. It is used in aromatherapy; its practitioners believe it to be a calming agent to reduce stress and aid in sleep.
- It can be used to create a fragrant chamomile lawn. A chamomile lawn needs light soil, adequate moisture, and sun to thrive. Each square meter contains 83-100 plants. The lawn is only suitable for light foot traffic or in places where mower access is difficult.

Chamomile health benefits:

- Improves overall skin health
- Relieves pain
- Aids sleep
- Reduces inflammation and swelling
- Rich source of antioxidants
- Relieves congestion

11. Centaury - Centaurium Ervtraea

What Is Centaury?

Centaury is a small, annual herb, native to Europe and naturalized in the United States. It thrives in boggy meadows as well as in dry dunes. The root is fibrous and woody. The plant has pale green, oval leaves, a capsule fruit, and light pink to red flowers. The whole herb is used in medicine. Synonyms are Erythraea Centaurium, C. umbellatum, C. minus. Centaurium consists of approximately 40 species (annuals or biennials).

What Is It Used For?

Traditional/Ethnobotanical uses

Genus Erythraea is derived from the Greek erythrose, relating to the red color of the flowers. The genus formerly was called Chironia, from Centaur, Chiron. Hippocrates describes Centaurium, under the Greek Kentareion and according to legend, Chiron (founder of medicine) used centaury to heal a wound inflicted by a poisoned arrow. Historically, centaury has been used as herbal medicine to kill worms, to treat dropsy, as a sedative, to treat snakebite and other wounds, and topically for freckles and spots. It is reputed to be an aromatic bitter and tonic for treating GI complaints such as bloating, dyspepsia, and flatulence, and anorexia. Centaury is said to act on the liver and kidneys to "purify the blood," and for jaundice. Centaury also was used traditionally to treat fever, hence the name "feverwort." This bitter herb enhances the production of gastric secretions, which stimulates appetite and improves digestion. Long-term use of the herb is required for the tonic effects on the stomach to fully develop. Other effects include anti-inflammatory as well as antimutagenic effects. Little research is available to support these traditional uses.

What Is The Recommended Dosage?

There is no recent published clinical evidence to guide dosage of the century. The German Commission E monograph calls for 1 to 2 g of herb daily, while other uses for dyspepsia specify as much as 6.

Contraindications

Contraindications have not yet been identified.

Pregnancy/Lactation

Information regarding safety and efficacy in pregnancy and lactation is lacking.

Interactions

None well documented.

Side Effects

There are no known adverse reactions.

Toxicology

There are no known reports of toxicity. Because the safety of centaury taken during pregnancy has not been established, its use during this time is best avoided.

12. Chaga - Inonotus Obliquus

Chaga is a fungus. It produces a woody growth, called a conk, which is used to make medicine. People take Chaga by mouth for heart disease, diabetes, stomach and intestine cancer, liver disease, parasites, stomach pain, and tuberculosis.

How Does It Work?

Chaga might stimulate the immune system. It contains some chemicals that have antioxidant effects. Chaga might lower blood sugar and cholesterol levels.

Uses & Effectiveness?

Insufficient Evidence For

- Heart disease.
- Diabetes.
- Gastritis.
- Stomach and intestinal cancer.
- Liver disease.
- Tuberculosis.
- Other conditions.

Side Effects & Safety

It isn't known if Chaga is safe or what the possible side effects might be. It contains a chemical called oxalate which can damage the kidneys.

Special Precautions & Warnings:

1. Pregnancy And Breast-Feeding: Not enough is known about the use of Chaga during pregnancy and breast-feeding. Stay on the safe side and avoid use.

2. Bleeding Disorders: There is concern that Chaga might increase the risk of bleeding. Don't use chaga if you have a bleeding disorder.

3. Diabetes: Chaga might lower blood sugar levels in people with diabetes. Watch for signs of low blood sugar (hypoglycemia) and monitor your blood sugar carefully if you have diabetes and use Chaga products. The dose of your diabetes medications may need to be adjusted by your healthcare provider.

4. Surgery: Chaga might affect blood sugar control or increase the risk of bleeding during and after surgery. Stop using Chaga at least 2 weeks before a scheduled surgery.

Dosing

The appropriate dose of Chaga depends on several factors such as the user's age, health, and several other conditions. At this time there is not enough scientific information to determine an appropriate range of doses for Chaga. Keep in mind that natural products are not always necessarily safe and dosages can be important. Be sure to follow relevant directions on product labels and consult your pharmacist or physician or other healthcare professional before using.

13. Chickweed - Stellaria Media

What Is Chickweed?

Chickweed is a common plant, particularly throughout Europe and North America. This low-growing annual has a thin hairy stem with pointed oval leaves. It produces small, white, star-shaped flowers throughout much of the year.

What Is It Used For?

Traditional/Ethnobotanical Uses

Chickweed has been used as a folk remedy for centuries for many conditions, including asthma, blood disorders, conjunctivitis, constipation, inflammation, dyspepsia, skin ailments, and obesity. Chickweed extract has been used internally as a demulcent but is more typically used externally for the treatment of rashes and sores. The young shoots are edible and have been used as salad greens. In homeopathy, the plant is used to relieve rheumatic pains and psoriasis. Chickweed is noted as a folk remedy for many conditions, including asthma, blood disorders, conjunctivitis, constipation, inflammation, dyspepsia, skin ailments, and obesity.

What Is The Recommended Dosage?

There is no recent published clinical evidence to guide the dosage of chickweed.

Contraindications

Contraindications have not yet been identified.

Pregnancy/Lactation

Information regarding safety and efficacy in pregnancy and lactation is lacking.

Interactions

None well documented.

Side Effects

Human cases of paralysis have been reported from large amounts of the infusion.

Toxicology

There is no overwhelming evidence to suggest that chickweed is toxic.

14. Damiana - Turnera Dif Usa Var. Aphrodisiac

What Is Damiana?

Damiana is a wild shrub that grows in Mexico, Central America, and the West Indies. The leaf and stem are used to make medicine. Historically, it was used mostly to increase sexual desire (as an aphrodisiac). Damiana is used to treat headaches, bedwetting, depression, nervous stomach, and constipation; for prevention and treatment of sexual problems; boosting and maintaining mental and physical stamina, and as an aphrodisiac. Some people inhale damiana for a slight "high."

Insufficient Evidence To Rate Effectiveness For

- Sexual problems
- Weight loss
- Headaches
- Bedwetting
- Depression
- Nervous upset stomach
- Constipation
- Boosting mental and physical stamina
- Other conditions.

How Does Damiana Work?

Damiana contains chemicals that may affect the brain and nervous system.

Are There Safety Concerns?

Damiana is LIKELY SAFE when taken by mouth in amounts commonly found in foods. Damiana is POSSIBLY SAFE when taken by mouth in medicinal amounts, but there have been serious side effects. Convulsions and other symptoms similar to rabies or strychnine poisoning have been reported after taking 200 grams of damiana extract.

Special Precautions & Warnings:

1. Pregnancy And Breast-Feeding: There is not enough reliable information about the safety of taking damiana if you are pregnant or breastfeeding. Stay on the safe side and avoid use.

2. Diabetes: Damiana might affect blood sugar levels in people with diabetes. Watch for signs of low blood sugar (hypoglycemia) and monitor your blood sugar carefully if you have diabetes and use damiana.

3. Surgery: Since damiana seems to affect blood glucose levels, there is a concern that it might interfere with blood glucose control during and after surgery. Stop using damiana at least 2 weeks before a scheduled surgery.

Are There Any Interactions With Medications?

1. Medications For Diabetes (Antidiabetes Drugs)Interaction Rating: Moderate Be cautious with this combination. Talk with your health provider.

2. Damiana Might Decrease Blood Sugar: Diabetes medications are also used to lower blood sugar. Taking damiana along with diabetes medications might cause your blood sugar to go too low. Monitor your blood sugar closely. The dose of your diabetes medication might need to be changed.

Some medications used for diabetes include glimepiride (Amaryl), glyburide (Diabeta, Glynase PresTabs, Micronase), insulin, metformin (Glucophage), pioglitazone (Actos), rosiglitazone (Avandia), and others.

Dosing Considerations For Damiana

The appropriate dose of damiana depends on several factors such as the user's age, health, and several other conditions. At this time there is not enough scientific information to determine an appropriate range of doses for damiana. Keep in mind that natural products are not always necessarily safe and dosages can be important. Be sure to follow relevant directions on product labels and consult your pharmacist or physician or other healthcare professional before using.

15. Dandelion - Taraxacum Of Icinale

Dandelion is an herb that is native to Europe. It is also found throughout mild climates of the northern hemisphere. People use dandelion for conditions such as swelling (inflammation) of the tonsils (tonsillitis), infections of the kidney, bladder, or urethra (urinary tract infections or UTIs), and many others, but there is no good scientific evidence to support these uses.

How Does It Work?

Dandelion contains chemicals that may increase urine production, prevent crystals from forming in the urine, and decrease swelling (inflammation).

Uses & Effcctiveness?

Insufficient Evidence For

- ❖ Arthritis-like pain.
- ❖ Bruises.
- ❖ Constipation.
- ❖ Eczema.
- ❖ Heart failure.
- ❖ Loss of appetite.
- ❖ Upset stomach.
- ❖ Intestinal gas (flatulence).
- ❖ Other conditions.

Side Effects & Safety

When taken by mouth: Dandelion is LIKELY SAFE for most people when taken by mouth in the amounts commonly found in food. It is POSSIBLY SAFE when taken by mouth in medicinal amounts (larger amounts than those found in food). Taking dandelion by mouth might cause allergic reactions, stomach discomfort, diarrhea, or heartburn in some people.

Special Precautions & Warnings:

1. Pregnancy And Breast-Feeding: There isn't enough reliable information to know if dandelion is safe to use when pregnant or breast-feeding. Stay on the safe side and avoid use.

2. Eczema: People with eczema seem to have a higher chance of having an allergic reaction to dandelion. If you have eczema, be sure to check with your healthcare provider before taking dandelion.

3. Bleeding Disorders: Dandelion might slow blood clotting. In theory, taking dandelion might increase the risk of bruising and bleeding in people with bleeding disorders.

4. Ragweed Allergy: People who are allergic to ragweed and related plants (daisies, chrysanthemums, marigolds) might be more likely to be allergic to dandelion. But conflicting data exists. If you have allergies, be sure to check with your healthcare provider before taking dandelion.

5. Kidney Failure: Dandelion might reduce how much oxalate is released through urine. In theory, this might increase the risk of complications in people with kidney problems.

Interactions

Moderate Interaction

Be cautious with this combination

1. Antibiotics (Quinolone Antibiotics) Interacts With DANDELION

Dandelion might decrease how much antibiotic the body absorbs. Taking dandelion along with antibiotics might decrease the effectiveness of some antibiotics. Some antibiotics that might interact with dandelion include ciprofloxacin (Cipro), enoxacin (Penetrex), norfloxacin (Chibroxin, Noroxin), sparfloxacin (Zagam), trovafloxacin (Trovan), and grepafloxacin (Raxar).

2. Lithium Interacts With DANDELION

Dandelion might affect a water pill or "diuretic." Taking dandelion might decrease how well the body gets rid of lithium. This could increase how much lithium is in the body and result in serious side effects. Talk with your healthcare provider before using this product if you are taking lithium. Your lithium dose might need to be changed. Medications changed by the liver (Cytochrome P450 1A2 (CYP1A2) substrates) interacts with DANDELION

3. Some Medications Are Changed And Broken Down By The Liver.

Dandelion might decrease how quickly the liver breaks down some medications. Taking dandelion along with some medications that are broken down by the liver can increase the effects and side effects of some medications. Before taking dandelion, talk to your healthcare provider if you take any medications that are changed by the liver.

4. Water Pills (Potassium-Sparing Diuretics) Interacts With DANDELION

Dandelion contains significant amounts of potassium. Some "water pills" can also increase potassium levels in the body. Taking some "water pills" along with dandelion might cause too much potassium to be in the body. Some "water pills" that increase potassium in the body include amiloride (Midamor), spironolactone (Aldactone), and triamterene (Dyrenium).

Dosing

The appropriate dose of dandelion depends on several factors such as the user's age, health, and several other conditions. At this time there is not enough scientific information to determine an appropriate range of doses for dandelion. Keep in mind that natural products are not always necessarily safe and dosages can be important. Be sure to follow relevant directions on product labels and consult your pharmacist or physician or other healthcare professional before using

16. Echinacea - Echinacea Angustifolia

What Is Echinacea?

Echinacea is an herb that is native to areas east of the Rocky Mountains in the United States. It is also grown in western States, as well as in Canada and Europe. Several species of the echinacea plant are used to make medicine from its leaves, flower, and root. Echinacea was used in traditional herbal remedies by the Great Plains Indian tribes. Later, settlers followed the Indians' example and began using echinacea for medicinal purposes as well. For a time, echinacea enjoyed official status as a result of being listed in the US National Formulary from 1916-1950. However, the use of echinacea fell out of favor in the United States with the discovery of antibiotics. But now, people are becoming interested in echinacea again because some antibiotics don't work as well as they used to against certain bacteria.

Echinacea is widely used to fight infections, especially the common cold, the flu, and other upper respiratory infections. Some people take echinacea at the first sign of a cold, hoping they will be able to keep the cold from developing. Other people take echinacea after cold symptoms have started, hoping they can make symptoms less severe.

Echinacea is also used against many other infections including urinary tract infections, vaginal yeast infections, herpes,

HIV/AIDS, human papillomavirus (HPV), bloodstream infections (septicemia), tonsillitis, streptococcus infections, syphilis, typhoid, malaria, ear infection, swine flu, warts, and nose and throat infections called diphtheria. Other uses include anxiety, low white blood cell count, chronic fatigue syndrome (CFS), rheumatoid arthritis, migraines, acid indigestion, pain, dizziness, rattlesnake bites, attention deficit-hyperactivity disorder (ADHD), and improving exercise performance.

Sometimes people apply echinacea to their skin to treat boils, gum disease, abscesses, skin wounds, ulcers, burns, eczema, psoriasis, sun-related skin damage, herpes simplex, yeast infections, bee stings, snake and mosquito bites, and hemorrhoids. Echinacea is also used as an injection to treat vaginal yeast infections and urinary tract infections (UTIs). Commercially available echinacea products come in many forms including tablets, juice, and tea.

There are concerns about the quality of some echinacea products on the market. Echinacea products are frequently mislabeled, and some may not even contain echinacea, despite label claims. Don't be fooled by the term "standardized." It doesn't necessarily indicate accurate labeling. Also, some echinacea products have been contaminated with selenium, arsenic, and lead.

Possibly Effective For

Common cold. Many scientific studies show that taking some echinacea products when cold symptoms are first noticed can modestly reduce symptoms of the common cold in adults. But other scientific studies show no benefit. The problem is that scientific studies have used different types of echinacea plants and different methods of preparation. Since the studies have not been consistent, it is not surprising that different studies show different results. If it helps for TREATING a cold, the benefit will likely be modest at best. Research on the effects of echinacea for PREVENTING the common cold is also mixed. Some research shows that taking echinacea can reduce the risk of catching a cold by 45% to 58%. But other research shows that taking echinacea does not prevent the common cold when you are exposed to cold viruses.

Insufficient Evidence To Rate Effectiveness For

1. Anxiety: Early research suggests that taking 40 mg of a specific echinacea extract (ExtractumPharma ZRT, Budapest, Hungary) per day for 7 days reduces anxiety. But taking less than 40 mg per day does not seem to be effective.

2. Exercise Performance: Early research shows that taking echinacea (Puritan's Pride, Oakdale, NY) four times daily for 28 days increases oxygen intake during exercise tests in healthy men.

3. Gingivitis: Early research suggests that using a mouth rinse containing echinacea, Gotu kola, and elderberry (HM-302, Izum Pharmaceuticals, New York, NY) three times daily for 14 days might prevent gum disease from worsening. Using a specific mouth patch containing the same ingredients (PerioPatch, Izun Pharmaceuticals, New York, NY) also seems to reduce some symptoms of gum disease, but it is not always effective.

4. Herpes Simplex Virus (HSV): Evidence on the effect of echinacea for the treatment of HSV is unclear. Some research shows that taking a specific echinacea extract (Echinaforce, A Vogel Bioforce AG) 800 mg twice daily for 6 months does not seem to prevent or reduce the frequency or duration of recurrent genital herpes. However, other research shows that taking a combination product containing echinacea (Esberitox, Schaper & Brummer, Salzgitter-Ringelheim, Germany) 3-5 times daily reduces itchiness, tension, and pain in most people with cold sores (herpes labialis).

5. Human Papillomavirus (HPV): Early research shows that taking a combination product containing echinacea, Andrographis, grapefruit, papaya, pau d'arco, and cat's claw (Immune Act, Erba Vita SpA, Reppublica San Marino, Italy) daily for one month reduces the recurrence of anal warts in people who had surgical removal of anal warts. But this study was not of high quality, so the results are questionable.

6. Influenza (Flu): Early research shows that taking a specific echinacea product (Monoselect Echinacea, PharmExtracta, Pontenure, Italy) daily for 15 days might improve the response to the flu vaccine in people with breathing problems such as bronchitis or asthma.

7. Middle Ear Infection: Early research suggests that taking a specific liquid echinacea extract three times daily for 3 days at the first sign of a common cold does not prevent ear infection in children 1-5 years-old with a history of ear infections. Ear infections seemed to increase.

8. Eye Inflammation (Uveitis): Early research suggests that taking 150 mg of an echinacea product (Iridium, SOOFT Italia SpA) twice daily, in addition to eye drops and a steroid used to treat inflammation for 4 weeks, does not improve vision any more than eye drops and steroids alone in people with eye inflammation.

How Does Echinacea Work?

Echinacea seems to activate chemicals in the body that decrease inflammation, which might reduce cold and flu symptoms. Laboratory research suggests that echinacea can stimulate the body's immune system, but there is no evidence that this occurs in people. Echinacea also seems to contain some chemicals that can attack yeast and other kinds of fungi directly.

Are There Safety Concerns?

Echinacea is LIKELY SAFE for most people when taken by mouth in the short-term. Various liquid and solid forms of Echinacea have been used safely for up to 10 days. There are also some products, such as Echinaforce (A. Vogel Bioforce AG, Switzerland) that have been used safely for up to 6 months.

Some side effects have been reported such as fever, nausea, vomiting, unpleasant taste, stomach pain, diarrhea, sore throat, dry mouth, headache, numbness of the tongue, dizziness, insomnia, disorientation, and joint and muscle aches. In rare cases, echinacea has been reported to cause inflammation of the liver.

Special Precautions & Warnings:

1. Children: Echinacea is POSSIBLY SAFE when taken by mouth in the short-term. It seems to be safe in most children ages 2-11 years. However, about 7% of these children may experience a rash that could be due to an allergic reaction. There is some concern that allergic reactions to echinacea could be more severe in some children. For this reason, some regulatory organizations have recommended against giving echinacea to children under 12 years of age.

2. Pregnancy: Echinacea is POSSIBLY SAFE when taken by mouth in the short-term. There is some evidence that echinacea might be safe when taken during the first trimester of pregnancy without harming the fetus. But until this is confirmed by additional research, it is best to stay on the safe side and avoid use.

3. Breastfeeding: There is not enough reliable information about the safety of taking echinacea if you are breastfeeding. Stay on the safe side and avoid use.

4. An Inherited Tendency Toward Allergies (Atopy): People with this condition are more likely to develop an allergic reaction to echinacea. It's best to avoid exposure to echinacea if you have this condition.

5. "Auto-immune disorders" such as multiple sclerosis (MS), lupus (systemic lupus erythematosus, SLE), rheumatoid arthritis (RA), a skin disorder called pemphigus Vulgaris or others: Echinacea might affect the immune system that could make these conditions worse. Don't take echinacea if you have an auto-immune disorder.

17. Feverfew - Chrysanthemum Parthenium

Feverfew is a plant that is native to Asia Minor and the Balkans. It is now commonly grown throughout the world. Feverfew leaves are normally dried for use in medicine. Fresh leaves and extracts are also used. People most commonly take feverfew by mouth for migraine headaches. People also take feverfew by mouth for itching, tension headache, and many other conditions, but there is no good scientific evidence to support these uses.

How Does It Work?

Feverfew leaves contain many different chemicals, including one called parthenolide. Parthenolide or other chemicals decrease factors in the body that might cause migraine headaches.

Uses & Effectiveness?

Possibly Effective For

1. Migraine: Some research using feverfew alone or feverfew combined with other ingredients shows that taking feverfew by mouth can reduce the frequency and duration of migraine headaches and might reduce pain, nausea, vomiting, and sensitivity to light and noise when they do occur. Feverfew may be more effective in people with more frequent migraine attacks.

Insufficient Evidence For

- Itching
- Tension headache
- Allergies
- Asthma
- Bone disorders
- Cancer

- Common cold
- Dizziness
- Earache
- Fever
- Intestinal parasites
- Liver disease
- Menstrual irregularities
- Miscarriage prevention
- Muscle tension
- Nausea
- Psoriasis
- Ringing in the ears
- Swollen feet
- Toothaches
- Upset stomach
- Vomiting
- Other conditions

Side Effects & Safety

1. When Taken By Mouth: Dried feverfew leaf or feverfew extract is LIKELY SAFE when taken by mouth appropriately in the short-term (up to 4 months). Side effects might include upset stomach, heartburn, diarrhea, constipation, bloating, flatulence, nausea, and vomiting. Other reported side effects include nervousness, dizziness, headache, trouble sleeping, joint stiffness, tiredness, menstrual changes, rash, pounding heart, and weight gain. The safety of feverfew beyond 4 months' use has not been studied. Feverfew is POSSIBLY UNSAFE when fresh leave is chewed. Chewing fresh feverfew leaves can cause mouth sores, swelling of the mouth, and loss of taste.

Special Precautions & Warnings

1. Pregnancy: Feverfew is POSSIBLY UNSAFE when taken by mouth during pregnancy. There is concern that it might cause early contractions and miscarriage. Don't use feverfew if you are pregnant.

2. Breast-Feeding: There is not enough reliable information about the safety of feverfew if you are breast-feeding. Stay on the safe side and avoid use.

3. Bleeding Disorders: Feverfew might slow blood clotting. In theory, taking feverfew could increase the risk of bleeding in some people. Until more is known, use feverfew cautiously if you have a bleeding disorder.

4. Allergy to ragweed and related plants: Feverfew may cause an allergic reaction in people who are sensitive to the Asteraceae/Compositae plant family. Members of this family include ragweed, chrysanthemums, marigolds, daisies, and many others. If you have allergies, be sure to check with your healthcare provider before taking feverfew.

5. Surgery: Feverfew might slow blood clotting. It might cause bleeding during and after surgery. Stop taking feverfew at least 2 weeks before a scheduled surgery.

Dosing

The following doses have been studied in scientific research:

1. **By Mouth:**

For migraine: 50-150 mg of feverfew powder taken once daily for up to 4 months. A dose of 2.08-18.75 mg of a carbon dioxide extract of feverfew (MIG-99, Schaper & Brümmer GmbH & Co) taken three times daily for 3 to 4 months.

The following combination products have been used for 3 months for preventing migraines: a combination of feverfew 300 mg and white willow 300 mg, taken twice daily (Mig-RL, Naturveda-Vitro-Bio Research Institute); a combination of feverfew 100 mg, coenzyme Q10, magnesium, and vitamin B6, taken daily (Antemig, PiLeJe); a combination of feverfew (containing Tanacetum parthenium 150 mg), 5-HTP, and magnesium, taken daily (Aurastop, Aesculapius Farmaceutici).

Specific combination products containing feverfew and ginger (GelStat Migraine, GelStat Corporation; LipiGesic M, PuraMed BioScience, Inc.) have been used to treat migraines after a migraine starts for up to 1 month. Two 2-mL doses have been given under the tongue, 5 minutes apart. Each dose has been held under the tongue for 60 seconds before swallowing.

18. Gravel Root - Eutrochium Purpureum

Gravel root is an herb. The bulb, root, and parts that grow above the ground are used to make medicine. Despite safety concerns, people use gravel root for conditions such as bladder infections, kidney stones, arthritis pain, fever, and many others, but there is no good scientific evidence to support these uses.

How Does It Work?

Gravel root might work for certain conditions by reducing swelling (inflammation).

Uses & Effectiveness?

Insufficient Evidence For

- Arthritis-like pain.
- Fever.
- Gout.
- Urinary and kidney stones.
- Urinary tract infections.
- Other conditions.

Side Effects & Safety

1. When Taken By Mouth: There's a lot of concern about using gravel root as medicine, because it contains chemicals called hepatotoxic pyrrolizidine alkaloids (PAs). These chemicals may block blood flow in the veins and cause liver or lung damage. Gravel root preparations that are not certified and labeled "hepatotoxic PA-free" are considered LIKELY UNSAFE. There isn't enough reliable information to know if it's safe to take "hepatotoxic PA-free" gravel root by mouth. It's best to avoid use.

2. When Applied To The Skin: It is LIKELY UNSAFE to apply gravel root to broken skin. The dangerous chemicals in gravel root can be absorbed quickly through broken skin and can lead to dangerous body-wide toxicity. Steer clear of skin products that aren't certified and labeled "hepatotoxic PA-free." There isn't enough reliable information to know if it's safe to apply "hepatotoxic PA-free" gravel root to the skin. It's best to avoid use.

Special Precautions & Warnings:

1. Pregnancy: It's LIKELY UNSAFE to use gravel root preparations that might contain hepatotoxic PAs during pregnancy. These products might cause birth defects and liver damage. It's not known whether products that are certified "hepatotoxic PA-free" are safe to use during pregnancy. Stay on the safe side and avoid using any gravel root preparation.

2. Breast-Feeding: It's LIKELY UNSAFE to use gravel root preparations that might contain hepatotoxic PAs if you are breast-feeding. These chemicals can pass into breast milk and might harm the nursing infant. It's not known whether products that are certified "hepatotoxic PA-free" are safe to use when breastfeeding. Stay on the safe side and avoid using any gravel root preparation.

3. Allergy To Ragweed And Related Plants: Gravel root may cause an allergic reaction in people who are allergic to the Asteraceae/Compositae plant family. Members of this family include ragweed, chrysanthemums, marigolds, daisies, and many others. If you have allergies, be sure to check with your healthcare provider before taking gravel root.

4. Liver Disease: There is concern that the hepatotoxic PAs in gravel root might make liver disease worse.

Dosing

The appropriate dose of gravel root depends on several factors such as the user's age, health, and several other conditions. At this time there is not enough scientific information to determine an appropriate range of doses for gravel root. Keep in mind that natural products are not always necessarily safe and dosages can be important. Be sure to follow relevant directions on product labels and consult your pharmacist or physician or other healthcare professional before using.

19. Hops - Humulus Lupulus

Hops are the dried, flowering part of the hop plant. They are commonly used in brewing beer and as flavoring components in foods. Hops are also used to make medicine. Hops are commonly used orally for anxiety, sleep disorders such as the inability to sleep (insomnia) or disturbed sleep due to rotating or nighttime work hours (shift work disorder), restlessness, tension, excitability, attention deficit-hyperactivity disorder (ADHD), nervousness, irritability, and symptoms of menopause among other uses. But there is limited scientific evidence to support using hopes for any of these conditions.

How Does It Work?

The chemicals in hops seem to have weak effects similar to the hormone estrogen. Some chemicals in hops also seem to reduce swelling, prevent infections, and cause sleepiness.

Uses & Effectiveness?

Insufficient Evidence For

- Anxiety
- Attention deficit-hyperactivity disorder (ADHD)
- Body odor
- Breast-feeding
- Breast cancer
- Excitability

- ❖ High levels of cholesterol or other fats (lipids) in the blood (hyperlipidemia)
- ❖ Improving appetite
- ❖ Indigestion (dyspepsia)
- ❖ Insomnia
- ❖ Intestinal cramps
- ❖ Irritability
- ❖ Leg sores are caused by weak blood circulation (venous leg ulcers)
- ❖ Nerve pain
- ❖ Nervousness
- ❖ Ovarian cancer
- ❖ Pain and swelling (inflammation) of the bladder
- ❖ Prostate cancer
- ❖ Restlessness
- ❖ Tension
- ❖ Tuberculosis

Side Effects & Safety

1. When Taken By Mouth: Hops are LIKELY SAFE when consumed in amounts commonly found in foods. Hops are POSSIBLY SAFE when taken for medicinal uses, short-term. Hops might cause dizziness and sleepiness in some people. Women taking hops might notice changes in their menstrual cycle.

Special Precautions & Warnings

1. **Pregnancy And Breast-Feeding:** There isn't enough reliable information to know if hops are safe to use when pregnant or breast-feeding. Stay on the safe side and avoid use.

2. **Depression:** Hops may make depression worse. Avoid use.

3. **Hormone-Sensitive Cancers And Conditions:** Some chemicals in hops act like the hormone estrogen. People who have conditions that are sensitive to hormones should avoid hops. Some of these conditions including breast cancer and endometriosis.

4. **Surgery:** Hops might cause too much sleepiness when combined with anesthesia and other medications during and after surgical procedures. Stop taking hops at least 2 weeks before a scheduled surgery.

Interactions?

Moderate Interaction

Alcohol Interacts With HOPS

Alcohol can cause sleepiness and drowsiness. Hops might also cause sleepiness and drowsiness. Taking large amounts of hops along with alcohol might cause too much sleepiness.

Dosing

The appropriate dose of hops depends on several factors such as the user's age, health, and several other conditions. At this time there is not enough scientific information to determine an appropriate range of doses for hops. Keep in mind that natural products are not always necessarily safe and dosages can be important. Be sure to follow relevant directions on product labels and consult your pharmacist or physician or other healthcare professional before using.

20. Mullein - Verbascum

What Is Mullein?

Mullein is a plant. The flower is used to make medicine. Mullein is used for cough, whooping cough, tuberculosis, bronchitis, hoarseness, pneumonia, earaches, colds, chills, flu, swine flu, fever, allergies, tonsillitis, and sore throat. Other uses include asthma, diarrhea, colic, gastrointestinal bleeding, migraines, joint pain, and gout. It is also used as a sedative and as a diuretic to increase urine output. Mullein is applied to the skin for wounds, burns, hemorrhoids, bruises, frostbite, and skin infections (cellulitis). The leaves are used topically to soften and protect the skin. In manufacturing, mullein is used as a flavoring ingredient in alcoholic beverages.

Insufficient Evidence To Rate Effectiveness For

- ❖ Ear infections (otitis media)
- ❖ Wounds
- ❖ Hemorrhoids

- ❖ Colds
- ❖ Flu
- ❖ Asthma
- ❖ Diarrhea
- ❖ Migraines
- ❖ Gout
- ❖ Tuberculosis
- ❖ Croup
- ❖ Cough
- ❖ Sore throat
- ❖ Inflammation of the airways (bronchitis)
- ❖ Other conditions

How Does Mullein Work?

The chemicals in mullein might be able to fight influenza and herpes viruses, and some bacteria that cause respiratory infections.

Are There Safety Concerns?

Mullein is POSSIBLY SAFE for when applied to the ear, short-term. A specific product (Otikon Otic Solution, Healthy-On Ltd.) that contains mullein, garlic, calendula, and St. John's wort has been used in the ear for up to 3 days.

Special Precautions & Warnings:

1. Children: Mullein is POSSIBLY SAFE when applied to the ear, short-term. A specific product (Otikon Otic Solution, Healthy-On Ltd.) that contains mullein, garlic, calendula, and St. John's wort has been used in the ear for up to 3 days.

2. Pregnancy And Breast-Feeding: There is not enough reliable information about the safety of taking mullein if you are pregnant or breast-feeding. Stay on the safe side and avoid use.

Dosing Considerations For Mullein

The appropriate dose of mullein depends on several factors such as the user's age, health, and several other conditions. At this time there is not enough scientific information to determine an appropriate range of doses for mullein. Keep in mind that natural products are not always necessarily safe and dosages can be important. Be sure to follow relevant directions on product labels and consult your pharmacist or physician or other healthcare professional before using.

21. Nettle - Urtica Dioica

Stinging Nettle

Stinging nettle is a plant. The root and above-ground parts are used as medicine. Stinging nettle is used for diabetes and osteoarthritis. It is sometimes used for urinary tract infections

(UTIs), kidney stones, enlarged prostate (benign prostatic hyperplasia or BPH), muscle pain, and other conditions, but there is no good scientific research to support these uses. In foods, young stinging nettle leaves are eaten as a cooked vegetable.

In manufacturing, stinging nettle extract is used as an ingredient in hair and skin products. Stinging nettle leaf has a long history of use. It was used primarily as a diuretic and laxative in ancient Greek times. Don't confuse stinging nettle (Urtica dioica) with white dead nettle (Lamium album).

How Does It Work?

Stinging nettle contains ingredients that might decrease inflammation and increase urine output.

Uses & Effectiveness?

Possibly Effective For

1. Diabetes: Taking stinging nettle leaf preparations for 8-12 weeks seems to reduce blood sugar in people with type 2 diabetes. The effect of stinging nettle on A1c in people with diabetes is unclear.

2. Osteoarthritis: Taking stinging nettle leaf preparations by mouth or applying it to the skin might reduce pain in people with osteoarthritis. Taking stinging nettle leaf preparations by mouth might also reduce the need for pain medications.

Insufficient Evidence For

- Hay fever
- A mild form of gum disease (gingivitis)
- Anemia
- Asthma
- Bleeding
- Cancer
- Diarrhea
- Eczema (atopic dermatitis)
- Heart failure
- Infections of the kidney, bladder, or urethra (urinary tract infections or UTIs)
- Joint pain
- Kidney stones
- Male-pattern baldness (androgenic alopecia)
- Muscle pai
- Poor circulation
- Rough, scaly skin on the scalp and face (seborrheic dermatitis)
- Water retention
- Wound healing
- Other conditions

Side Effects & Safety

1. When Taken By Mouth: Stinging nettle is POSSIBLY SAFE when taken by mouth for up to 2 years. It might cause diarrhea, constipation, and upset stomach in some people.

2. When Applied To The Skin: Stinging nettle is POSSIBLY SAFE when applied to the skin in appropriate amounts. Touching the stinging nettle plant can cause skin irritation.

Special Precautions & Warnings:

1. Pregnancy And Breast-Feeding: Stinging nettle is LIKELY UNSAFE to take during pregnancy. It might stimulate uterine contractions and cause a miscarriage. It's also best to avoid stinging nettle if you are breast-feeding.

2. Diabetes: There is some evidence that stinging nettle above-ground parts can decrease blood sugar levels. This might increase the chance of blood sugar levels becoming too low in people being treated for diabetes. Monitor your blood sugar carefully.

3. Low Blood Pressure: Stinging nettle above ground parts might lower blood pressure. In theory, stinging nettle might increase the risk of blood pressure dropping too low in people prone to low blood pressure. If you have low blood pressure, discuss stinging nettle with your healthcare provider before starting it.

4. Kidney Problems: The above-ground parts of stinging nettle seem to increase urine flow. If you have kidney problems, discuss stinging nettle with your healthcare provider before starting it.

Dosing

The following doses have been studied in scientific research:

Adults

By Mouth:

1. For Diabetes: 500 mg of stinging nettle leaf extract has been taken three times per day for 12 weeks. Also, 3.3 grams of stinging nettle leaf has been taken three times daily for 8 weeks. A combination product containing 200 mg of stinging nettle, 200 mg of milk thistle, and 200 mg of frankincense taken three times per day for 3 months has also been used.

2. For Osteoarthritis: 9 grams of crude stinging nettle leaf has been used daily. Also, an infusion containing 50 mg of stinging nettle leaf has been taken along with 50 mg of diclofenac daily for 14 days.

Applied To The Skin:

For osteoarthritis: Fresh stinging nettle leaf has been applied to painful joints for 30 seconds once per day for one week. Also, a specific cream containing stinging nettle leaf extract (Liquid

Phyto-Caps Nettle Leaf by Gaia Herbs) has been applied twice daily for 2 weeks.

22. Oregon Grape - Mahonia Aquifolium

The Oregon grape (Mahonia aquifolium) is a broadleaf evergreen shrub that grows well in shadier spots. It originated in western North America and is the state flower of Oregon. It will provide color throughout all four seasons with its green and burgundy foliage, yellow flowers, and purplish-blue fruit.

Hardiness And Growing Tips

The soil needs to be moist with good drainage for optimal growth. It needs to be acidic or at least neutral as alkaline soils can be problematic. Change your soil to be more acidic if the pH is not too much above neutral.

This shrub is best suited for USDA Zones 5-9. It is native to western North America. Partial shade is ideal for this species. It can also be grown in full shade or full sun, though too much light can cause foliage scorching. Try to find a planting location that offers some shelter from the wind. Since these are evergreen and do not drop in the fall, the leaves may dry out in the winter if the shrub is hit by wind often.

Propagation can be performed through the use of seed germination, taking cuttings, and dividing existing plants. The plant will also naturally propagate itself through cloning.

Size And Design Tips

Oregon grape will be 3 to 10 feet tall and 2 to 5 feet wide. Look for the 'Compactum' cultivar if you want a shrub that is shorter, at 3 feet tall. Or, if you want a similar looking shrub that is more of a groundcover, choose the creeping mahonia (Mahonia repens). This species only is about a foot tall at maturity.

The fruit is a berry that does resemble a grape in shape and color. They are edible but are quite tart and can be used to make jams, jellies, and preserves. Oregon grape can be used as part of a wildlife garden to attract butterflies, bees, hummingbirds, and other birds to your yard.

This shrub can clone itself and spread. On one hand, this can be a useful feature as you can use it to populate a native garden or divide to create new plants. However, this tendency can also lead to the species being invasive in some locations. Your local extension service will know if it is a problem in your area.

Foliage

The evergreen leaves are sharply toothed like members of the holly genus as noted in the species name. It can be used as a privacy screen to keep unwanted visitors out since the leaves are sharp. These are pinnately compound leaves that are up to 12" long and made up of several leaflets. When they first appear, they are red. As time passes they turn into a shiny green hue. During autumn, they become burgundy but do not fall off.

Health Benefits

The root of Oregon grape has been used as herbal medicine to treat many maladies including colds, flu, herpes, hepatitis, syphilis, stomach upset, cancer, skin disorders, yeast infections, and more. Herbalists have touted the use of Oregon grape, claiming that it is effective in stimulating liver function, treating infections, and supporting digestive health.

It's important to note that there are limited clinical research study results available on the safety and health benefits of the Oregon grape. Most of the published clinical research study results on Oregon grape involved the use of the root of the herb in a topical (administered on the skin) cream, for the treatment of a skin condition called psoriasis. Oregon grape has also been used for its digestive stimulant properties (relieving spasms in the intestinal tract), antimicrobial properties (including its anti-fungal, antibacterial, and anti-parasitic action), immune-boosting, and anti-inflammatory properties.

Medical Uses

Oregon grape has been demonstrated to help lower blood sugar in patients with insulin resistance. It also has some cholesterol-lowering effects. The herb has traditionally been used for maladies including, eye infections, acne, athlete's foot, gastrointestinal issues, skin conditions, and more, though there is limited scientific research on these claims.

Some studies have shown that Oregon grape may be effective for the treatment of giardia (a type of infectious diarrhea), eczema (an inflammatory skin condition), and as an herbal treatment for urinary tract infections. The primary medicinal component of Oregon grape, berberine, has been shown to have anti-bacterial properties that are helpful in the treatment of several infections including, throat, intestinal, and urinary tract infections. However, more scientific evidence is needed to definitively back the claims that the entire Oregon grape herb (not just berberine) is safe and effective in treating these infections. Extensive medical research data has shown that Oregon grape may be safe and effective for the treatment of psoriasis (a common skin condition that causes skin cells to form scales and itchy, sometimes painful red patches).

23. Primrose (Evening) Oil - Oenothera Biennis

Evening primrose is a plant native to North and South America. It also grows throughout Europe and parts of Asia. It has yellow flowers which open at sunset and close during the day. The oil from the seeds of evening primrose is used to make medicine. Evening primrose is used for premenstrual syndrome (PMS), symptoms of menopause, arthritis, swelling, and other conditions, but there is no good scientific evidence to support its use. In foods, the oil from evening primrose is used as a source of essential fatty acids. In manufacturing, the oil from evening primrose is used in soaps and cosmetics.

How Does It Work?

Evening primrose oil contains "fatty acids." Some women with breast pain might not have high enough levels of certain "fatty acids." Fatty acids also seem to help decrease inflammation related to conditions such as arthritis and eczema.

Uses & Effectiveness?

Possibly Effective For

1. Nerve Damage Caused By Diabetes: Research shows that taking evening primrose oil daily for 6-12 months improves symptoms of nerve damage caused by diabetes.

2. Osteoporosis: Taking evening primrose oil with fish oil and calcium seems to decrease bone loss and increase bone density in elderly people with osteoporosis.

Possibly Ineffective For

1. Asthma: Several small studies show that taking 15-20 mL or 4-6 grams of evening primrose daily for up to 16 weeks doesn't improve asthma symptoms.

2. Breast Pain (Mastalgia): High-quality research shows that evening primrose is no more effective than a placebo (sugar pill) for reducing breast pain.

Insufficient Evidence For

1. Eczema (Atopic Dermatitis): Research evaluating evening primrose for eczema shows conflicting results. Some research shows that taking evening primrose, up to 6 grams per day by mouth for 3-5 months, reduces the severity and symptoms of eczema in adults and children. However, other studies show that taking evening primrose, 6-8 grams per day in adults or 2-4 grams per day in children for 12-16 weeks, has no benefit. Other early research shows that applying a cream containing evening primrose for 2 weeks may improve symptoms of eczema.

2. Chronic Fatigue Syndrome (CFS): One early study shows that taking a specific combination of evening primrose and fish oil might reduce CFS-like symptoms that occurred after a viral infection. However, in another study in people with a confirmed diagnosis of CFS, the same product was no better than a placebo (sugar pill).

3. Nerve Pain In People With Diabetes (Diabetic Neuropathy): Evidence on the effectiveness of evening primrose for treating nerve damage in people with diabetes is conflicting. One study shows that taking up to 6 grams of evening primrose daily for up to 12 months improves how well the nerves work in people with nerve damage caused by diabetes. Other research shows that taking a similar amount of evening primrose does not improve nerve function in people with this condition.

4. Dry Eye: Early research shows that taking a specific evening primrose product 3 grams daily for 6 months improves dry eye symptoms in women wearing soft contact lenses.

5. Swelling (inflammation) of the liver caused by the hepatitis B virus (hepatitis B). Early research shows that taking 4 grams per day of evening primrose for 12 months does not improve liver damage in people with hepatitis B.

6. High levels of cholesterol or other fats (lipids) in the blood (hyperlipidemia). Some research shows that taking evening primrose oil can decreases total cholesterol and blood fats called triglycerides while increasing good (HDL) cholesterol. But not all research agrees.

7. An inherited skin disorder that causes dry, scaly skin (ichthyosis). Early research shows that taking evening primrose, 3 grams per day in adults or 2 grams per day in children, does not improve symptoms of ichthyosis.

8. Liver Cancer: Early research shows that taking 18 grams of evening primrose per day does not affect liver size or survival in people with liver cancer.

9. Symptoms Of The Menopause: In most studies, taking evening primrose does not reduce hot flashes or night sweats any more than a placebo (sugar pill). But taking evening primrose oil might help to improve mood.

10. Multiple Sclerosis (MS): Some early research shows that taking evening primrose for 6 months improves disability scores in some people with MS. But other research shows that using a specific evening primrose product for 2 years may increase the likelihood of symptom worsening compared with a placebo (sugar pill).

11. Childbirth: However, another study did not show this effect. Other early research shows that taking evening primrose from week 37 of pregnancy until delivery doesn't improve childbirth. It might prolong labor and increase the need for contraction-inducing medicine (oxytocin).

12. Rheumatoid Arthritis (RA): One early study shows that taking 6 grams per day of evening primrose for 12 months improves self-reported symptoms of RA. However, other research has found evening primrose to be no better than a placebo (sugar pill).

- ❖ A motor skill disorder marked by clumsiness (developmental coordination disorder or DCD).
- ❖ Water warts.
- ❖ Diabetes.
- ❖ A learning disorder marked by difficulty reading (dyslexia).

- ❖ Low bone mass (osteopenia).
- ❖ A hormonal disorder that causes enlarged ovaries with cysts (polycystic ovary syndrome or PCOS).
- ❖ Scaly, itchy skin (psoriasis).
- ❖ Joint swelling (inflammation) in people with psoriasis.
- ❖ A type of inflammatory bowel disease (ulcerative colitis).
- ❖ Alzheimer disease.
- ❖ Heart disease.
- ❖ Infant development.
- ❖ Schizophrenia.
- ❖ Other conditions.

Side Effects & Safety

1. When Taken By Mouth: Evening primrose is LIKELY SAFE for most people when taken by mouth in doses up to 6 grams daily. It may cause mild side effects including upset stomach, nausea, diarrhea, and headache in some people.

2. When Applied To The Skin: Evening primrose is LIKELY SAFE for most people when applied to the skin.

Special Precautions & Warnings

1. Pregnancy And Breast-Feeding: Taking evening primrose by mouth is POSSIBLY SAFE during pregnancy. Taking up to 4 grams daily for up to 10 weeks during pregnancy seems to be safe. But until this is confirmed by additional research, it is best to stay on the safe side and avoid use. Taking evening primrose during the last weeks of pregnancy might delay labor. Don't use this product close to the end of pregnancy.

2. Children: Evening primrose is LIKELY SAFE for most people when taken by mouth in doses up to 6 grams daily. It is also LIKELY SAFE when applied to the skin.

3. Bleeding Disorders: There is a concern that evening primrose might increase the chance of bruising and bleeding. Don't use it if you have a bleeding disorder.

4. Epilepsy Or Another Seizure Disorder: There is a concern that taking evening primrose might make seizures more likely in some people.

5. Schizophrenia: Seizures have been reported in people with schizophrenia treated with phenothiazine drugs, GLA (a chemical found in evening primrose oil), and vitamin E. Get your healthcare provider's opinion before starting evening primrose.

6. Surgery: Evening primrose might increase the chance of bleeding during or after surgery. Stop using it at least 2 weeks before a scheduled surgery.

Dosing

The following doses have been studied in scientific research:

By Mouth:

For breast pain: 3-4 grams daily.

24. Purslane - Portulaca Oleracea

Purslane

Use

Purslane has been used as a vegetable source of omega-3 fatty acids and is high in vitamins and minerals. It possesses marked antioxidant activity. Roles in abnormal uterine bleeding, asthma, type 2 diabetes, and oral lichen planus are suggested; however, clinical studies are limited and diverse.

Dosing

Limited clinical studies are available to provide dosage guidelines; however, 180 mg/day of purslane extract has been studied in diabetic patients, and powdered seeds have been taken at 1 to 30 g daily in divided doses, as well as both ethanol and aqueous purslane extracts. Traditional Chinese Medicine recommendations of 9 to 15 g of dried aerial parts, and 10 to 30 g fresh herb, have been reported for a variety of indications. One hundred grams of fresh purslane leaves yields approximately 300 to 400 mg of alpha-linolenic acid.

Contraindications

Contraindications have not been identified.

Pregnancy/Lactation

Information regarding safety and efficacy in pregnancy and lactation is lacking.

Interactions

None well documented.

Adverse Reactions

Limited clinical studies have not reported clinically important adverse effects. Effects on uterine contractions are contradictory.

Health Benefits Of Purslane

Health Benefits Nutrition How To Eat Purslane

Purslane, also known as little hogweed, is a common weed worldwide. But just because it's considered a weed doesn't mean it's worthless. This salty, slightly sour plant, is completely edible and provides some impressive health benefits. Purslane is a succulent that offers a juicy bite. This allows it to be grown in conditions that would kill even the hardiest lettuce. Its sturdy nature makes purslane a great garden-vegetable option for dry, hot regions or gardeners who don't trust themselves to water regularly. Purslane's health benefits are an added benefit for this hearty, gardener's treasure.

Health Benefits

Purslane has vitamins, minerals, and antioxidants that can provide important health benefits. For example, vitamin A helps your eyes remain healthy as well as improve your immune system. Vitamin A is also critical to the health of your organs because it supports healthy cell division. Purslane is also rich in vitamin C, which is important to keep your collagen and blood vessels in good shape, as well as helping injuries heal.

Also, Purslane Can Provide Other Health Benefits, Like:

1. **Lower Risk Of Cancer**

Purslane is full of beta-carotene, the pigment responsible for the reddish color of its stems and leaves. Beta-carotene is one of many antioxidants s found in purslane. These antioxidants have been found to reduce the number of free radicals in your body. Free radicals are oxygen by-products given off by all cells in the body. Lowering the number of free radicals can help reduce the risk of cellular damage. This, in turn, lowers your risk of cancer.

2. **Heart Health**

Purslane is also helpful for supporting your cardiovascular system. It is one of the few vegetables that are rich in omega-3 fatty acids, which are important to support healthy arteries and can help prevent strokes, heart attacks, and other forms of heart disease. Purslane has the highest recorded levels of omega-3 fatty acids of any land-based plant.

3. Bone Health

Purslane is also a great source of two minerals that are important to bone health: calcium and magnesium. Calcium is the most common mineral in your body, and failing to eat enough of it can slowly weaken your bones, leading to osteoporosis. On the other hand, magnesium indirectly affects skeletal health by affecting the growth of bone cells. Getting enough of both of these minerals can improve skeletal health and prevent complications from osteoporosis and aging.

Nutrition

Purslane is rich in folate, which aids in safe cell division and promotes DNA duplication. Doctors recommend that people who can become pregnant consume at least 400 mcg of folate daily because it helps avoid birth defects.

Purslane is also an excellent source of:

- ❖ Vitamin A
- ❖ Vitamin C
- ❖ Potassium
- ❖ Calcium
- ❖ Iron

- Folate
- Choline
- Magnesium

How To Eat Purslane

Purslane can easily be found outdoors during the spring and summer in most parts of the world. The plant reproduces easily and can survive harsh growing environments, so it's often spotted between cracks in the sidewalk or untended gardens. Any purslane plant can be harvested and eaten, as the leaves, stems, and flowers are completely edible. When preparing wild purslane, it's important to wash the plant carefully to ensure that no pesticides are on the leaves. Purslane is tart and a little salty, making it a great addition to salads and other dishes. It can be eaten raw or cooked. When added to soups and stew, it thickens the broth nicely.

Here Are Some Ways You Can Include Purslane In Your Diet:

- Add purslane to soups
- Sauté purslane as a side dish
- Chop purslane and add it to salads for color
- Mix purslane into grilled vegetables
- Use purslane as a garnish
- Sprinkle purslane flowers on fish as a point of interest

25. Passionflower - Passiflora Incarnata

Passionflower is a climbing vine that is native to the southeastern United States, and Central and South America. The above-ground parts are used to make medicine. Passionflower is used for anxiety, including anxiety before surgery. Some people take passionflower for insomnia, stress, attention deficit-hyperactivity disorder (ADHD), pain, and many other conditions. But there is no good scientific research to support these uses. In foods and beverages, passionflower extract is used as a flavoring.

How does it work?

The chemicals in passionflower have to calm, sleep-inducing, and muscle spasm relieving effects. Passionflower is a climbing vine that is native to the southeastern United States, and Central and South America. The above-ground parts are used to make medicine.

Uses & Effectiveness?

Possibly Effective For

1. Anxiety: Some research shows that taking passion flower by mouth can reduce symptoms of anxiety. It might work as effectively as some prescription medications.

2. Anxiety Before Surgery: Some research shows that taking passion flower by mouth can reduce anxiety before surgery when taken 30-90 minutes before surgery. It might work as effectively as some other treatments for pre-operative anxiety such as melatonin or midazolam.

Insufficient Evidence For

- Attention deficit-hyperactivity disorder (ADHD)
- Insomnia
- Alcohol use disorder
- Asthma
- Burns
- Diarrhea
- Fibromyalgia
- Heart failure and fluid build up in the body (congestive heart failure or CHF)
- Hemorrhoids
- Inability to cope or adjust to a stressful event (adjustment disorders)
- Indigestion (dyspepsia)
- Irregular heartbeat (arrhythmia).
- Menstrual cramps (dysmenorrhea)
- Muscle cramps
- Pain
- Premenstrual syndrome (PMS)
- Seizures are not caused by epilepsy
- Stress
- Symptoms of the menopause

❖ Other conditions

Side Effects & Safety

1. When Taken By Mouth: Passionflower is LIKELY SAFE for most people when used in food-flavoring amounts. It is POSSIBLY SAFE for most people when taken as a tea nightly for 7 nights, or as a medicine for up to 8 weeks. It may cause side effects such as drowsiness, dizziness, and confusion.

It is POSSIBLY UNSAFE for most people when taken by mouth in large amounts, such as 3.5 grams of a specific extract (Sedacalm by Bio plus Healthcare) over 2 days.

2. When Applied To The Skin: There isn't enough reliable information to know if passionflower is safe or what the side effects might be when applied to the skin.

Special Precautions & Warnings:

1. Children: Passionflower is POSSIBLY SAFE for most children when taken by mouth for short periods. A specific passionflower product (Pasipay by Iran Darouk Pharmaceutical Company) has been used safely in children aged 6-13 years at a dose of 0.04 mg per kg body weight daily for up to 8 weeks.

2. Pregnancy: Passionflower is POSSIBLY UNSAFE when taken by mouth during pregnancy. There are some reports of early labor and other problems when passionflower has been used in pregnancy. There are some chemicals in the passionflower plant that might cause the uterus to contract. Don't use passionflower if you are pregnant.

3. Breast-feeding: There isn't enough reliable information to know if passionflower is safe to use when breastfeeding. Stay on the safe side and avoid use.

4. Surgery: Passionflower might cause drowsiness. It might increase the effects of anesthesia and other medications on the brain during and after surgery. Talk to your healthcare provider if you are taking passion flower within 2 weeks of scheduled surgery.

Dosing

The following doses have been studied in scientific research:

Adults

By Mouth:

1. For Anxiety: Capsules containing 400 mg of passionflower extract twice daily for 2-8 weeks has been used. Also, 45 drops of a liquid extract of passionflower have been used daily for up to one month.

2. For Reducing Anxiety Before Surgery: 20 drops of a specific passionflower extract taken the evening before surgery and 90 minutes before the start of surgery has been used. Passionflower 260-1000 mg has been taken 30-90 minutes before dental surgery. Also, a syrup containing 700 mg of passionflower extract (Passiflora syrup by Sandoz) has been taken 30 minutes before surgery.

26. Red Clover - Trifolium Pratense

Red clover is a plant. The flowers are used to make medicine. Red clover is used for symptoms of menopause, weak and brittle bones, high levels of cholesterol, and many other conditions, but there is no good scientific evidence to support these uses. In foods and beverages, red clover is used as a flavoring ingredient. Red clover (Trifolium pratense) is an herb that belongs to the legume family, which also includes peas and beans. In herbal medicine, red clover is typically used to treat respiratory issues (such as asthma, whooping cough, and bronchitis), skin disorders (such as eczema and psoriasis), inflammatory conditions like arthritis, and women's health problems1 (such as menopausal and menstrual symptoms).

Red clover's brightly colored flowers contain many nutrients including calcium, chromium, magnesium, niacin, phosphorus, potassium, thiamine, and vitamin C. They're also a rich source of isoflavones. These are compounds that act as phytoestrogens plant chemicals similar to the female hormone estrogen. Isoflavone extracts are touted as dietary supplements for high cholesterol and osteoporosis in addition to menopausal symptoms.

Health Benefits

In alternative medicine, red clover is said to help with the following conditions. Note, however, that research hasn't shown that the herb is conclusively effective for these or any other health concerns.

1. Menopausal Symptoms

Several small studies have been done to see if red clover may help relieve the discomforts of menopause, especially hot flashes. Though you may hear some anecdotal support for this, there has been no conclusive evidence to back it up. A research review conducted in 2013 notes that phytoestrogen treatments (including red clover) are not proven to effectively alleviate menopausal symptoms.

2. Bone Loss

Research is ongoing as to whether isoflavones lower the loss of bone mineral density in postmenopausal women. Red clover is one source of supplements used in some studies. A review done in 2016 concluded there may be some beneficial effects on bone health, while a 2017 review found that different formulations of red clover may be effective or ineffective.

3. Cancer

Preliminary research suggests that red clover may help reduce the risk of prostate cancer. In a 2009 study of prostate cancer cells, scientists found that treatment with red clover led to a decrease in the prostate-specific antigen (PSA), a protein found at elevated levels in men with prostate cancer.

4. Heart Disease

A few clinical trials have looked at the effects of red clover on the development of risk factors for heart disease in postmenopausal women, with no strong evidence that it helps, reports Memorial Sloan Kettering Cancer Center. Keep in mind that, due to the lack of long-term studies, it's too soon to recommend red clover for any condition. It's also important to note that self-treating a condition and avoiding or delaying standard care may have serious consequences.

5. Selection And Preparation

Red clover is available in a variety of preparations, including teas, tinctures, tablets, capsules, liquid extract, and extracts standardized to specific isoflavone contents. It's not always clear, however, that a product contains the promised isoflavone content.

Making Red Clover Tea

You can also make tea from dried flower heads. Some proponents claim that to get the full benefit of red clover you need to use the whole flower, and not commercial red clover isoflavones, which many studies use. To make a tea, use one to three teaspoons of dried red clover flowers for every cup of simmering (not boiling) water. Let steep for 15 minutes. Drink up to three cups of tea a day.

How Does It Work?

Red clover contains chemicals called phytoestrogens that are similar to the hormone estrogen.

Uses & Effectiveness?

Possibly Ineffective For

Weak and brittle bones (osteoporosis). Most research shows that taking red clover daily does not improve the density of bones in women.

Insufficient Evidence For

1. Male-Pattern Baldness (Androgenic Alopecia): Early research shows that applying a combination product containing red clover flower extract might increase hair growth in people with hair loss.

2. Enlarged Prostate (Benign Prostatic Hyperplasia Or BPH): Some early research suggests that red clover supplements might improve some symptoms of an enlarged prostate. It seems to reduce nighttime urination.

3. Breast Pain (Mastalgia): There is some early evidence that red clover might help relieve cyclic breast pain and tenderness.

4. High Cholesterol: Most research shows that taking red clover extracts by mouth for 3 months to a year does not seem to reduce low-density lipoprotein (LDL or "bad") cholesterol or increase high-density lipoprotein (HDL or "good") cholesterol in women who have moderately elevated cholesterol levels.

- Symptoms of the menopause.
- Asthma.
- Eczema (atopic dermatitis).
- Breast cancer.
- Swelling (inflammation) of the main airways in the lung (bronchitis).
- Burns.
- Cough.
- Indigestion (dyspepsia).Cancer of the lining of the uterus (endometrial cancer).
- Premenstrual syndrome (PMS).
- Sexually transmitted diseases (STDs).
- Scaly, itchy skin (psoriasis).
- Whooping cough (pertussis).
- Wound healing.

Side Effects & Safety

1. When Taken By Mouth: Red clover is LIKELY SAFE for most people when used in the amounts found in food. It is POSSIBLY SAFE when used in medicinal amounts. Red clover can cause rashes, muscle aches, headache, nausea, and vaginal bleeding (spotting) in some women.

2. When Applied To The Skin: Red clover is POSSIBLY SAFE when applied in medicinal amounts.

Special Precautions & Warnings:

1. Pregnancy And Breast-Feeding: Red clover is LIKELY SAFE when taken by mouth in amounts commonly found in food. However, it is LIKELY UNSAFE when used in medicinal amounts. Red clover acts like estrogen and might disturb important hormone balances during pregnancy or breast-feeding. Don't use it.

2. Bleeding Disorders: Red clover might increase the chance of bleeding. Avoid large amounts and use with caution.

3. Protein S Deficiency: People with protein S deficiency have an increased risk of forming blood clots. There is some concern that red clover might increase the risk of clot formation in these people because it has some of the effects of estrogen. Don't use red clover if you have protein S deficiency.

4. Surgery: Red clover might slow blood clotting. It might increase the chance of bleeding during and after surgery. Stop taking red clover at least 2 weeks before a scheduled surgery.

Dosing

The appropriate dose of red clover depends on several factors such as the user's age, health, and several other conditions. At this time there is not enough scientific information to determine an appropriate range of doses for red clover. Keep in mind that natural products are not always necessarily safe and dosages can be important. Be sure to follow relevant directions on product labels and consult your pharmacist or physician or other healthcare professional before using

27. Sassafras Sassafras Albidum

What Is Sassafras?

Sassafras is a plant. The root bark is used to make medicine. Despite serious safety concerns, sassafras is used for urinary tract disorders, swelling in the nose and throat, syphilis, bronchitis, high blood pressure in older people, gout, arthritis, skin problems, and cancer. It is also used as a tonic and "blood purifier." Some people apply sassafras directly to the skin to treat skin problems, achy joints (rheumatism), swollen eyes, sprains, and insect bites or stings. Sassafras oil is also applied to the skin to kill germs and head lice.

In beverages and candy, sassafras was used in the past to flavor root beer. It was also used as a tea. But sassafras tea contains a lot of safrole, the chemical in sassafras that makes it poisonous. One cup of tea made with 2.5 grams of sassafras contains about 200 mg of safrole.

Insufficient Evidence To Rate Effectiveness For

- Urinary tract problems
- Gout
- Arthritis
- Skin problems
- Eye swelling
- Sprains
- Insect bites and stings
- Purifying the blood

How Does Sassafras Work?

There isn't enough information available to know how sassafras works.

Are There Safety Concerns?

Sassafras seems safe in foods and beverages if it is "safrole-free."

However, it is UNSAFE for use as a medicine. Don't take it by mouth or put it on your skin. The safrole in sassafras root bark and oil can cause cancer and liver damage. Consuming just 5 mL of sassafras oil can kill an adult. Even "safrole-free" sassafras used in medicinal amounts has been linked with tumors. Sassafras can cause sweating and hot flashes. High amounts can cause vomiting, high blood pressure, hallucinations, and more severe side effects. It can cause skin rashes when used on the skin.

Special Precautions & Warnings:

It is UNSAFE for anyone to use sassafras in medicinal amounts, but some people have extra reasons not to use it:

1. Pregnancy And Breast-Feeding: Don't use sassafras if you are pregnant. There is evidence that sassafras oil might cause a miscarriage.

2. Children: Sassafras is UNSAFE for children. A few drops of sassafras oil may be deadly.

3. Surgery: In medicinal amounts, sassafras can slow down the central nervous system. This means it can cause sleepiness and drowsiness. When combined with anesthesia and other medications used during and after surgery, it might slow down the central nervous system too much. Stop using sassafras at least 2 weeks before a scheduled surgery.

4. Urinary Tract Conditions: Sassafras might make these conditions worse.

Are There Any Interactions With Medications?

Sedative medications (CNS depressants)Interaction Rating: Moderate Be cautious with this combination. Talk with your health provider.

Sassafras might cause sleepiness and drowsiness. Medications that cause sleepiness are called sedatives. Taking sassafras along with sedative medications might cause too much sleepiness.

Some sedative medications include clonazepam (Klonopin), lorazepam (Ativan), phenobarbital (Donnatal), zolpidem (Ambien), and others.

Dosing Considerations For Sassafras.

The appropriate dose of sassafras depends on several factors such as the user's age, health, and several other conditions. At this time there is not enough scientific information to determine an appropriate range of doses for sassafras. Keep in mind that natural products are not always necessarily safe and dosages can be important. Be sure to follow relevant directions on product labels and consult your pharmacist or physician or other healthcare professional before using.

28. Skullcup Scutellaria Lateriflora

Skullcap is a plant. The above-ground parts are used to make medicine. Skullcap is used for many conditions, but so far, there isn't enough scientific evidence to determine whether or not it is effective for any of them. Skullcap is used for trouble sleeping (insomnia), anxiety, stroke, and paralysis caused by stroke. It is also used for fever, high cholesterol, "hardening of the arteries" (atherosclerosis), rabies, epilepsy, nervous tension, allergies, skin infections, inflammation, and spasms.

Skullcap products are not always what the labels claim. The plant's germander and teucrium are often unwanted and unlabeled ingredients in skullcap products. Secondly, you may think you are buying Scutellaria lateriflora, the species of skullcap that has been studied for medicinal use, but the product may contain a different species of skullcap instead. The most often substituted species are Western Skullcap (Scutellaria canescens), Southern Skullcap (Scutellaria cordifolia), or Marsh Skullcap (Scutellaria galericulatum). These species contain different chemicals, so they are not considered interchangeable.

How Does It Work?

The chemicals in the skullcap might work by preventing swelling (inflammation). Other chemicals in the skullcap are thought to cause sedation (drowsiness).

Uses & Effectiveness?

Insufficient Evidence For

- ❖ Anxiety.

- ❖ Seizures.
- ❖ Trouble sleeping (insomnia).
- ❖ Stroke.

Side Effects & Safety

There is not enough information available to know if a skullcap is safe to take for medical conditions.

Special Precautions & Warnings

1. Pregnancy And Breast-Feeding: There is not enough reliable information about the safety of taking a skullcap is you are pregnant or breastfeeding. Stay on the safe side and avoid use.

2. Surgery: Skullcap may slow down the central nervous system. Healthcare providers worry that anesthesia and other medications during and after surgery might increase this effect. Stop taking skullcap at least 2 weeks before a scheduled surgery.

Dosing

The appropriate dose of skullcap depends on several factors such as the user's age, health, and several other conditions. At this time there is not enough scientific information to determine an appropriate range of doses for skullcap. Keep in mind that natural products are not always necessarily safe and dosages can be important. Be sure to follow relevant directions on product labels and consult your pharmacist or physician or other healthcare professional before using.

29. Turkey Corn Dicentra Canadensis

What Is Turkey Corn?

Turkey corn is a plant. The fleshy root (tuber) is used to make medicine. Despite serious safety concerns, people take turkey corn for digestion problems, urinary tract diseases, and skin rashes. Women take it for menstrual disorders.

Insufficient Evidence To Rate Effectiveness For

- ❖ Digestive problems.
- ❖ Menstrual disorders.
- ❖ Urinary tract diseases.
- ❖ Skin rashes.

How Does Turkey Corn Work?

Turkey corn might help the body get rid of extra fluids by increasing urine production.

Are There Safety Concerns?

Turkey corn seems to be UNSAFE. It may cause poisoning.

Special Precautions & Warnings

Pregnancy and breast-feeding: Since turkey corn seems to be UNSAFE, it's best to avoid use, especially if you are pregnant or breast-feeding.

Are There Any Interactions With Medications?

1. Lithium Interaction Rating: Moderate Be cautious with this combination. Talk with your health provider.

2. Turkey corn might affect a water pill or "diuretic." Taking turkey corn might decrease how well the body gets rid of lithium. This could increase how much lithium is in the body and result in serious side effects. Talk with your healthcare provider before using this product if you are taking lithium. Your lithium dose might need to be changed.

Dosing Considerations For Turkey Corn

The appropriate dose of turkey corn depends on several factors such as the user's age, health, and several other conditions. At this time there is not enough scientific information to determine an appropriate range of doses for turkey corn. Keep in mind that natural products are not always necessarily safe and dosages can be important. Be sure to follow relevant directions on product labels and consult your pharmacist or physician or other healthcare professional before using.

30. Valerian - Valeriana Officinalis

What Is Valerian?

Valerian is an herb. Medicine is made from the root. Valerian is most commonly used for sleep disorders, especially the inability to sleep (insomnia). It is frequently combined with hops, lemon balm, or other herbs that also cause drowsiness. Some people who are trying to withdraw from the use of "sleeping pills" use valerian to help them sleep after they have tapered the dose of the sleeping pill. There is some scientific evidence that valerian works for sleep disorders, although not all studies are positive. Valerian is also used for conditions connected to anxiety and psychological stress including nervous asthma, hysterical states, excitability, fear of illness (hypochondria), headaches, migraine, and stomach upset.

Some people use valerian for depression, mild tremors, epilepsy, attention deficit-hyperactivity disorder (ADHD), and chronic fatigue syndrome (CFS). Valerian is used for muscle and joint pain. Some women use valerian for menstrual cramps and symptoms associated with menopause, including hot flashes and anxiety. Sometimes, valerian is added to bathwater to help with restlessness and sleep disorders. In manufacturing, the extracts and oil made from valerian are used as a flavoring in foods and beverages.

Is Valerian Effective?

There is some scientific evidence that valerian can help people who have trouble sleeping. It seems to help people fall asleep faster and get a better night's rest. Valerian might work about as well as some low-dose sleeping pills, but it may take up to a month of nightly use before sleeping improves. There is also some evidence that valerian can improve mood and the ability to concentrate.

There isn't enough information to know whether or not valerian is effective for the other conditions people use it for, including depression, convulsions, mild tremors, epilepsy, attention-deficit hyperactivity disorder (ADHD), muscle and joint pain, headache, stomach upset, menstrual pains, menopausal symptoms including hot flashes and anxiety, and many others. Do not use valerian for these conditions until more is known.

Possibly Effective For

Inability to sleep (insomnia). Some research suggests that valerian does not relieve insomnia as fast as "sleeping pills." Continuous use for several days, even up to four weeks, maybe needed before an effect is noticeable. Valerian seems to improve the sleep quality of people who are withdrawing from the use of sleeping pills. Not all evidence is positive, however. Some studies have found that valerian doesn't improve insomnia any better than a "sugar pill" (placebo).

Insufficient Evidence To Rate Effectiveness For

- Anxiety
- Depression
- Restlessness
- Menstrual disorders (dysmenorrhea)
- Stress
- Convulsions
- Mild tremors
- Epilepsy
- Attention-deficit hyperactivity disorder (ADHD)
- Chronic fatigue syndrome (CFS)
- Muscle and joint pain
- Headache
- Stomach upset
- Menopausal symptoms including hot flashes and anxiety.

How Does Valerian Work?

Valerian seems to act as a sedative on the brain and nervous system.

Are There Safety Concerns?

Valerian can cause some side effects such as headache, excitability, uneasiness, and even insomnia in some people. A few people feel sluggish in the morning after taking valerian, especially at higher doses. It's best not to drive or operate dangerous machinery after taking valerian. The long-term safety of valerian is unknown. To avoid possible side effects when discontinuing valerian after long-term use, it's best to reduce the dose slowly over a week or two before stopping completely.

Special Precautions & Warnings

1. Pregnancy Or Breast-Feeding: There isn't enough information about the safety of valerian during pregnancy or breast-feeding. Stay on the safe side and avoid use.

2. Surgery: Valerian slows down the central nervous system. Anesthesia and other medications used during surgery also affect the central nervous system. The combined effects might be harmful. Stop taking valerian at least two weeks before a scheduled surgery.

Are There Any Interactions With Medications?

AlcoholInteraction Rating: Major Do Not Take This Combination.

Alcohol can cause sleepiness and drowsiness. Valerian might also cause sleepiness and drowsiness. Taking large amounts of valerian along with alcohol might cause too much sleepiness. However, some research has found that combining valerian with alcohol does not increase sleepiness.

Alprazolam (Xanax)Interaction Rating: Moderate Be cautious with this combination. Talk with your health provider.

Valerian can decrease how quickly the liver breaks down alprazolam (Xanax). Taking valerian with alprazolam (Xanax) might increase the effects and side effects of alprazolam (Xanax) such as drowsiness.

Some medications are changed and broken down by the liver. Valerian might decrease how quickly the liver breaks down some medications. Taking valerian along with some medications that are broken down by the liver can increase the effects and side effects of some medications. Before taking valerian, talk to your healthcare provider if you are taking any medications that are changed by the liver.

Sedative medications (Benzodiazepines)Interaction Rating: Moderate Be cautious with this combination. Talk with your health provider.

Valerian might cause sleepiness and drowsiness. Drugs that cause sleepiness and drowsiness are called sedatives. Taking valerian along with sedative medications might cause too much sleepiness.

Some of these sedative medications include alprazolam (Xanax), clonazepam (Klonopin), diazepam (Valium), lorazepam (Ativan), midazolam (Versed), temazepam (Restoril), triazolam (Halcion), and others.

Sedative medications (CNS depressants)Interaction Rating: Moderate Be cautious with this combination. Talk with your health provider.

Some sedative medications include pentobarbital (Nembutal), phenobarbital (Luminal), secobarbital (Seconal), thiopental (Pentothal), fentanyl (Duragesic, Sublimaze), morphine, propofol (Diprivan), and others.

Some medications are changed and broken down by the liver. Valerian might decrease how quickly the liver breaks down some medications. Taking valerian along with some medications that are broken down by the liver can increase the effects and side effects of some medications. Before taking valerian, talk to your healthcare provider if you are taking any medications that are changed by the liver.

Dosing Considerations For Valerian.

The following doses have been studied in scientific research:

By Mouth:

For The Inability To Sleep (Insomnia):

- ❖ 400-900 mg valerian extract up to 2 hours before bedtime for as long as 28 days, or
- ❖ Valerian extract 120 mg, with lemon balm extract 80 mg 3 times daily for up to 30 days, or

- A combination product containing valerian extract 187 mg plus hops extract 41.9 mg per tablet, 2 tablets at bedtime for 28 days.
- Take valerian 30 minutes to 2 hours before bedtime.

31. Wormwood - Artemisia Absinthium

What Is Wormwood?

Wormwood is an herb. The above-ground plant parts and oil are used for medicine. Wormwood is used for various digestion problems such as loss of appetite, upset stomach, gall bladder disease, and intestinal spasms. Wormwood is also used to treat fever, liver disease, and worm infections; to increase sexual desire; as a tonic; and to stimulate sweating. Wormwood oil is also used for digestive disorders, to increase sexual desire, and to stimulate the imagination. Some people apply wormwood directly to the skin for healing wounds and insect bites. Wormwood oil is used as a counterirritant to reduce pain. In manufacturing, wormwood oil is used as a fragrance component in soaps, cosmetics, and perfumes. It is also used as an insecticide.

Wormwood is used in some alcoholic beverages. Vermouth, for example, is a wine beverage flavored with extracts of wormwood. Absinthe is another well-known alcoholic beverage made with wormwood. It is an emerald-green alcoholic drink that is prepared from wormwood oil, often along with other dried herbs such as anise and fennel. Absinthe was popularized by famous artists and writers such as Toulouse-Lautrec, Degas, Manet, van Gogh, Picasso, Hemingway, and Oscar Wilde. It is now banned in many countries, including the U.S. But it is still allowed in European Union countries as long as the thujone content is less than 35 mg/kg. Thujone is a potentially poisonous chemical found in wormwood. Distilling wormwood in alcohol increases the thujone concentration.

Insufficient Evidence To Rate Effectiveness For

- Loss of appetite
- Indigestion
- Gallbladder disorders
- Wounds
- Insect bites
- Worm infestations
- Low sexual desire
- Spasms
- Increasing sweating

How Does Wormwood Work?

Wormwood oil contains the chemical thujone, which excites the central nervous system. However, it can also cause seizures and other adverse effects.

Are There Safety Concerns?

Wormwood is LIKELY SAFE when taken by mouth in the amounts commonly found in food and beverages including bitters and vermouth, as long as these products are thujone-free. Wormwood that contains thujone is POSSIBLY UNSAFE when it is taken by mouth. Thujone can cause seizures, muscle breakdown (rhabdomyolysis), kidney failure, restlessness, difficulty sleeping, nightmares, vomiting, stomach cramps, dizziness, tremors, urine retention, thirst, numbness of arms and legs, paralysis, and death.

Special Precautions & Warnings

1. Pregnancy And Breast-Feeding: Wormwood is LIKELY UNSAFE when taken by mouth during pregnancy in amounts greater than what is commonly found in food. The concern is the possible thujone content. Thujone might affect the uterus and endanger the pregnancy. It's also best to avoid topical wormwood since not enough is known about the safety of applying wormwood directly to the skin. If you are breast-feeding, don't use wormwood until more is known about safety.

2. Allergy To Ragweed And Related Plants: Wormwood may cause an allergic reaction in people who are sensitive to the Asteraceae/Compositae family. Members of this family include ragweed, chrysanthemums, marigolds, daisies, and many others. If you have allergies, be sure to check with your healthcare provider before taking wormwood.

3. A Rare Inherited Blood Condition Called Porphyria: Thujone present in wormwood oil might increase the body's production of chemicals called porphyrins. This could make porphyria worse.

4. Kidney Disorders: Taking wormwood oil might cause kidney failure. If you have kidney problems, talk with your healthcare provider before taking wormwood.

5. Seizure Disorders, Including Epilepsy: Wormwood contains thujone, which can cause seizures. There is concern that wormwood might make seizures more likely in people who are prone to them.

Are There Any Interactions With Medications?

Medications used to prevent seizures (Anticonvulsants)Interaction Rating: Moderate Be cautious with this combination. Talk with your health provider.

Medications used to prevent seizures affect chemicals in the brain. Wormwood may also affect chemicals in the brain. By affecting chemicals in the brain, wormwood may decrease the effectiveness of medications used to prevent seizures.

Some medications used to prevent seizures include phenobarbital, primidone (Mysoline), valproic acid

(Depakene), gabapentin (Neurontin), carbamazepine (Tegretol), phenytoin (Dilantin), and others.

Dosing Considerations For Wormwood

The appropriate dose of wormwood depends on several factors such as the user's age, health, and several other conditions. At this time there is not enough scientific information to determine an appropriate range of doses for wormwood. Keep in mind that natural products are not always necessarily safe and dosages can be important. Be sure to follow relevant directions on product labels and consult your pharmacist or physician or other healthcare professional before using.

32. Witch Hazel Hamamelis Virginiana

Witch hazel is a plant. The leaf, bark, and twigs are used to make medicine. You may see a product called witch hazel water (Hamamelis water, distilled witch hazel extract). This is a liquid that is distilled from dried leaves, bark, and partially dormant twigs of witch hazel. Witch hazel is taken by mouth for diarrhea, mucus colitis, vomiting blood, coughing up blood, tuberculosis, colds, fevers, tumors, and cancer.

Some people apply witch hazel directly to the skin for itching, pain, and swelling (inflammation), eye inflammation, skin injury, mucous membrane inflammation, vaginal dryness after menopause, varicose veins, hemorrhoids, bruises, insect bites, minor burns, acne, sensitive scalp, and other skin irritations. In manufacturing, witch hazel leaf extract, bark extract, and witch hazel water are used as astringents to tighten the skin. They are also included in some medications to give those products the ability to slow down or stop bleeding. Those medications are used for treating insect bites, stings, teething, hemorrhoids, itching, irritations, and minor pain.

How Does It Work?

Witch hazel contains chemicals called tannins. When applied directly to the skin, witch hazel might help reduce swelling, help repair broken skin, and fight bacteria.

Uses & Effectiveness?

Possibly Effective For

1. Hemorrhoids: Applying witch hazel water to the skin may help to temporarily relieve itching, discomfort, irritation, and burning from hemorrhoids and other anal disorders.

2. Minor Bleeding: Applying witch hazel bark, leaf, or water to the skin reduces minor bleeding.

3. Skin Irritation: Applying witch hazel cream seems to relieve mild skin irritation, but not as well as hydrocortisone. Other research shows that applying a specific witch hazel ointment (Hametum) to the skin appears to improve symptoms of skin injury or irritated skin as effectively as a dexpanthenol ointment in children.

Possibly Ineffective For

1. Itchy And Inflamed Skin (Eczema): Applying a cream containing witch hazel to the skin for 14 days does not seem to improve itchy and inflamed skin in people with moderate eczema. Applying hydrocortisone cream seems to be a more effective treatment option.

Insufficient Evidence For

- Health problems after menopause.
- Bruises.
- Colds.
- Coughing up blood.
- Diarrhea.
- Eye inflammation.
- Fevers.
- Tuberculosis.
- Varicose veins.
- Vomiting blood.

Side Effects & Safety

Witch hazel is LIKELY SAFE for most adults when applied directly to the skin. In some people, it might cause minor skin irritation. Witch hazel is POSSIBLY SAFE for most adults when small doses are taken by mouth. In some people, witch hazel might cause stomach upset when taken by mouth. Large doses might cause liver problems. Witch hazel contains a cancer-causing chemical (safrole), but in amounts that are too small to be of concern.

Special Precautions & Warnings

1. Children: Witch hazel is POSSIBLY SAFE for children when applied directly to the skin.

2. Pregnancy And Breast-Feeding: There is not enough reliable information about the safety of taking witch hazel if you are pregnant or breast-feeding. Stay on the safe side and avoid use.

Dosing

The following doses have been studied in scientific research:

Adults

Applied To The Skin:

For Skin Irritation: An after sun lotion containing 10% witch hazel water has been used.

Applied To The Anus:

For itching and discomfort associated with hemorrhoids and other anal disorders: Witch hazel water has been applied up to

6 times per day or after every bowel movement. Suppositories have been placed in the anus 1-3 times per day.

Children

Applied To The Skin:

For Skin Irritation: An ointment containing witch hazel has been applied several times per day in children aged 2-11 years.

CONCLUSION

As our lifestyle is now getting techno-savvy, we are moving away from nature. While we cannot escape from nature because we are part of nature. As herbs are natural products they are free from side effects, they are comparatively safe, eco-friendly, and locally available. Traditionally there are a lot of herbs used for ailments related to different seasons. There is a need to promote them to save human lives.

Medicinal plants are useful to keep on hand to treat common ailments. You can reach for certain medical plants to relieve headaches, tummy trouble, and even irritation from bug bites. Plants can be consumed in teas, used as a garnish, applied topically as an essential oil, or consumed as a pill.

These herbal products are today are the symbol of safety in contrast to the synthetic drugs, that are regarded as unsafe to human being and environment. Although herbs had been priced for their medicinal, flavoring, and aromatic qualities for centuries, the synthetic products of the modern age surpassed their importance, for a while. However, the blind dependence on synthetics is over and people are returning to the naturals with the hope of safety and security. It's time to promote them globally.

Medicinal plants, also called medicinal herbs, have been discovered and used in traditional medicine practices since prehistoric times. Plants synthesize hundreds of chemical compounds for functions including defense against insects, fungi, diseases, and herbivorous mammals. Numerous phytochemicals with potential or established biological activity have been identified. However, since a single plant contains widely diverse phytochemicals, the effects of using a whole plant as medicine are uncertain. Further, the phytochemical content and pharmacological actions, if any, of many plants having medicinal potential remain unassessed by rigorous scientific research to define efficacy and safety. It's important to remember that you should always double-check with your doctor before consuming or using anything new for your body. If you choose to grow some of these plants, remember to take proper care according to the plant's care guidelines and refrain from using any pesticides or other harmful chemicals on your plants. You don't want any of those chemicals in or on your body!

NATIVE AMERICAN HERBAL DISPENSATORY

Natural Herbal Remedies, Sacred Medicinal Plants, and Recipes to Heal Common Ailments

Taahira Maskwa

INTRODUCTION

Plants, herbs, and ethnobotanicals have been used since the early days of humankind and are still used throughout the world for health promotion and treatment of disease. Plants and natural sources form the basis of today's modern medicine and contribute largely to the commercial drug preparations manufactured today. About 25% of drugs prescribed worldwide are derived from plants. Still, herbs, rather than drugs, are often used in health care. For some, herbal medicine is their preferred method of treatment.

For others, herbs are used as an adjunct therapy to conventional pharmaceuticals. However, in many developing societies, the traditional medicine of which herbal medicine is a core part is the only system of health care available or affordable. Regardless of the reason, those using herbal medicines should be assured that the products they are buying are safe and contain what they are supposed to, whether this is a particular herb or a particular amount of a specific herbal component.

Consumers should also be given science-based information on dosage, contraindications, and efficacy. To achieve this, global harmonization of legislation is needed to guide the responsible production and marketing of herbal medicines. If sufficient scientific evidence of benefit is available for an herb, then such legislation should allow for this to be used appropriately to promote the use of that herb so that these benefits can be realized for the promotion of public health and the treatment of disease.

Health care is moving into the home increasingly often and involving a mixture of people, a variety of tasks, and a broad diversity of devices and technologies; it is also occurring in a range of residential environments. The factors driving this migration include the rising costs of providing health care; the growing numbers of older adults; the increasing prevalence of chronic disease; improved survival rates of various diseases, injuries, and other conditions (including those of fragile newborns); large numbers of veterans returning from war with serious injuries; and a wide range of technological innovations. The health care that results varies considerably in its safety, effectiveness, and efficiency, as well as it's quality and cost.

Results show that traditional medicine, and especially self-treatment with medicinal plants, prevail as treatment options in both rural and peri-urban populations. Contrary to what is commonly assumed, high income is an important determinant of the use of traditional medicine. Likewise, knowledge of medicinal plants, age, education, gender, and illness chronicity were also significant determinants. The importance of self-treatment with medicinal plants should inform the development of health policy tailored to people's treatment-seeking behavior.

High income and knowledge of medicinal plants are important determinants of the use of traditional medicine. This challenges the common assumption that poor and marginalized people are most reliant on traditional medicine due to its availability. Future health policies shall consider the high reliance on self-treatment and the importance of knowledge held within the household about this

Although many issues related to home health care could not be addressed, applications of human factors principles, knowledge, and research methods in these areas could make home health care safer and more effective and also contribute to reducing costs. The committee chose not to prioritize the recommendations, as they focus on various aspects of health care in the home and are of comparable importance to the different constituencies affected.

Background: The use of herbal products in children is a concern because little information is available concerning the benefits and risks of these products in the pediatric population.

Objective: This article defines herbal products and reviews the reasons for using such products, the most commonly used herbal products in the United States, their use during pregnancy and breast-feeding, and the adverse effects, drug interactions, and regulatory issues associated with herbal products.

Methods: A literature search was conducted using MEDLINE and references from journal articles.

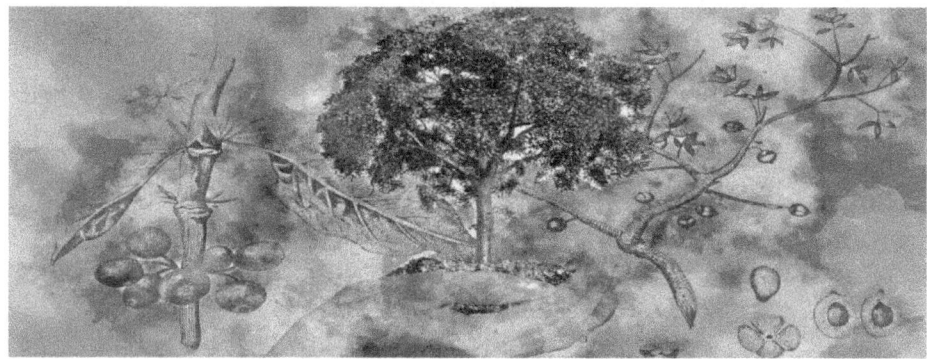

CHAPTER 1 : NATIVE AMERICAN TRADITIONS

Native American traditions, religious beliefs, and sacramental practices of the indigenous peoples of North and South America. Until the 1950s it was commonly assumed that the religions of the surviving Native Americans were little more than curious anachronisms, dying remnants of humankind's childhood. These traditions lacked sacred texts and fixed doctrines or moral codes and were embedded in societies without wealth, mostly without writing, and without recognizable systems of politics or justice or any of the usual indicators of civilization. Today the situation has changed dramatically. Scholars of religion, students of the ecological sciences, and individuals committed to expanding and deepening their own religious lives have found in these traditions many distinct and varied religious worlds that have struggled to survive but that retain the ability to inspire.

Native American people themselves often claim that their traditional ways of life do not include "religion." They find the term difficult, often impossible, to translate into their languages. This apparent incongruity arises from differences in cosmology and epistemology. Western tradition distinguishes religious thought and action as that whose ultimate authority is supernatural—which is to say, beyond, above, or outside both phenomenal nature and human reason. In most indigenous worldviews there is no such antithesis. Plants and animals, clouds, and mountains carry and embody revelation. Even where native tradition conceives of a realm or world apart from the terrestrial one and not normally visible from it, as in the case of the Iroquois Sky World or the several underworlds of Pueblo cosmologies, the boundaries between these worlds are permeable. The ontological distance between land and sky or between land and underworld is short and is traversed in both directions.

Instead of encompassing a duality of sacred and profane, indigenous religious traditions seem to conceive only of sacred and more sacred. Spirit, power, or something akin moves in all things, though not equally. For native communities religion is understood as the relationship between living humans and other persons or things, however, they are conceived. These may include departed as well as yet-to-be-born human beings, beings in the so-called "natural world" of flora and fauna, and visible entities that are not animate by Western standards, such as mountains, springs, lakes, and clouds. This group of entities also includes what scholars of religion might denote as "mythic beings," beings that are not normally visible but are understood to inhabit and affect either this world or some other world contiguous to it.

Spirituality And Connection

Before delving into more specific information about what native peoples believed, it makes sense to explain that the concept of religion as an organized thing is not a part of most traditions. Religion describes a division between the supernatural, which is ruled by one or multiple deities. Instead of calling their beliefs and practices a set religion, most refer to it as a system of spirituality that permeates every aspect of their lives. Religion is a set doctrine of supernatural beliefs, the ceremonies, and activities associated with it, and includes things like concepts of deities, spirits, or ghosts, what happens to a person after death, and certain special occasions throughout a person's life.

Native American spirituality includes similar ideas, but integrates them more into everyday living rather than reserving them for special occasions. Of course, there are ceremonies for births, deaths, marriages, harvests, and other special times, but daily life was just as filled with beliefs as "holidays" would be. Native American spirituality does not separate the two concepts in any real way. The spiritual or supernatural world is the same thing as the real world. Every supposed division is completely permeable and people can access everything spiritual just as easily as they can wade in a river or feel the sun on their skin.

There also exists a general sense of connection and oneness among a particular tribe of Native American people. The Lakota term "mitakuye oyasin" means that all are related or all beings are relations of each other.[ii] This explains the belief that spirit exists in everything or that everything is connected ins some ways. This does not necessarily encompass an objectified spiritual connection because the concept behind the phrase also pushes for respect for the individual.

Misunderstandings about the purpose behind the word, especially in non-native and non-Lakota communities, carry quite a bit of conflict. Still, the idea that all people and things are part of a whole and should respect and honor each other is not damaging in any way.

No concepts of unattainability or inaccessibility seem to exist for many Native American belief systems. Everything exists about everything else. This concept leads to the belief that tribal people are "one with nature" or similar ideas. Although phrases like that are often used in New Age philosophies, it does, at its core, also pertain to this idea of the spiritual existing firmly in the realm of tangible reality.

Healers

Native American (NA) traditional healing is identified by the National Institutes of Health/National Center for Complementary and Alternative Medicine (NCCAM) as a whole medical system that encompasses a range of holistic treatments used by indigenous healers for a multitude of acute and chronic conditions or to promote health and wellbeing.2 While there are individual tribal differences (i.e., the use of specific healing practices), there are also shared health beliefs and interventional strategies, including a health promotion foundation that embraces bio-psycho-socio-spiritual approaches and traditions. For thousands of years, traditional indigenous medicine has been used to promote health and wellbeing for millions of Native people who once inhabited this continent. Native diets, ceremonies that greet the seasons and the harvests, and the use of native plants for healing purposes have been used to live to promote health by living in harmony with the earth.

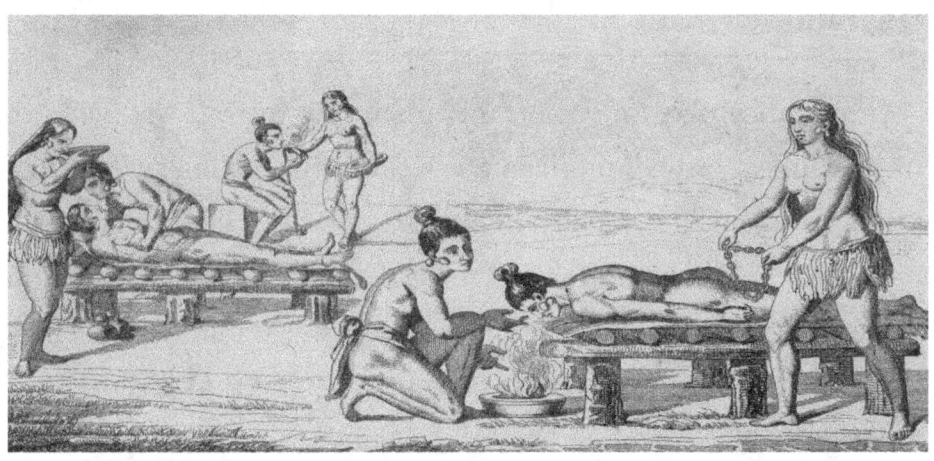

Today Native Americans frequently combine traditional healing practices with allopathic medicine to promote health and wellbeing. The ceremony, native herbal remedies, and allopathic medications are used side by side. Spiritual treatments are thus an integral part of health promotion and healing in Native American culture.

Yet, the role of spirituality in health promotion and wellness is uncomfortable for many allopathic providers. Advanced practice nurses with their tradition of holism that embraces the bio-psycho-social-spiritual nature of health have an opportunity to suggest new ways to care modeled on traditional NA practices. The inclusion of family and community in treatment plans decreases the isolation often found in allopathic care. And, thinking about the lack of person-environment harmony and balance may important clues for the diagnostic process.

Symbolic Healing

Ceremonies play an important role in the overall wellbeing of traditional Native American people but the healing potential of this practice is typically unappreciated by allopathic health providers. NA ceremonies involve the patient, the family, and the community in the healing process. Ceremonial gatherings may last for days or weeks; the more people that are present, the greater the healing energy. Through their participation in songs, prayer, music, and dance, the family and community contribute healing energy to the patient.

People of all cultures utilize symbolism found in their various religions and spiritual practices to cope with health problems. NA healing ceremonies rely heavily on a combination of traditional and Christian religious symbols, icons, and ritualistic objects. These symbols cue bio-psycho-social-spiritual healing responses by restoring the harmony necessary for health. Symbolism, whether associated with ceremonies or church services, can be incorporated into their treatment plan to create a powerful healing synergy.3

Healing And Ceremony

Many healing practices and spiritual ceremonies that are being practiced today by healing practitioners and metaphysical groups have been adopted from traditions that originated from various Native American tribes. History indicates that each tribe would have one or more elders who were groomed in the healing arts. These individuals would serve as herbalists, healers, and spirit communicators. The duties and types of healing arts and spiritual ceremonies performed would naturally vary from tribe to tribe. Native American healing arts and practices are earth-based, honoring and respectful of the Father Sky, Mother Earth, Grandfather Sun, and Grandmother Moon.

The ceremony is an essential part of traditional Native healing. Because physical and spiritual health is intimately connected, body and spirit must heal together. Traditional healing ceremonies promote wellness by reflecting Native conceptions of Spirit, Creator, and the Universe. They can include prayer, chants, drumming, songs, stories, and the use of a variety of sacred objects. Healers may conduct ceremonies anywhere a sick person needs healing, but ceremonies are often held in sacred places.

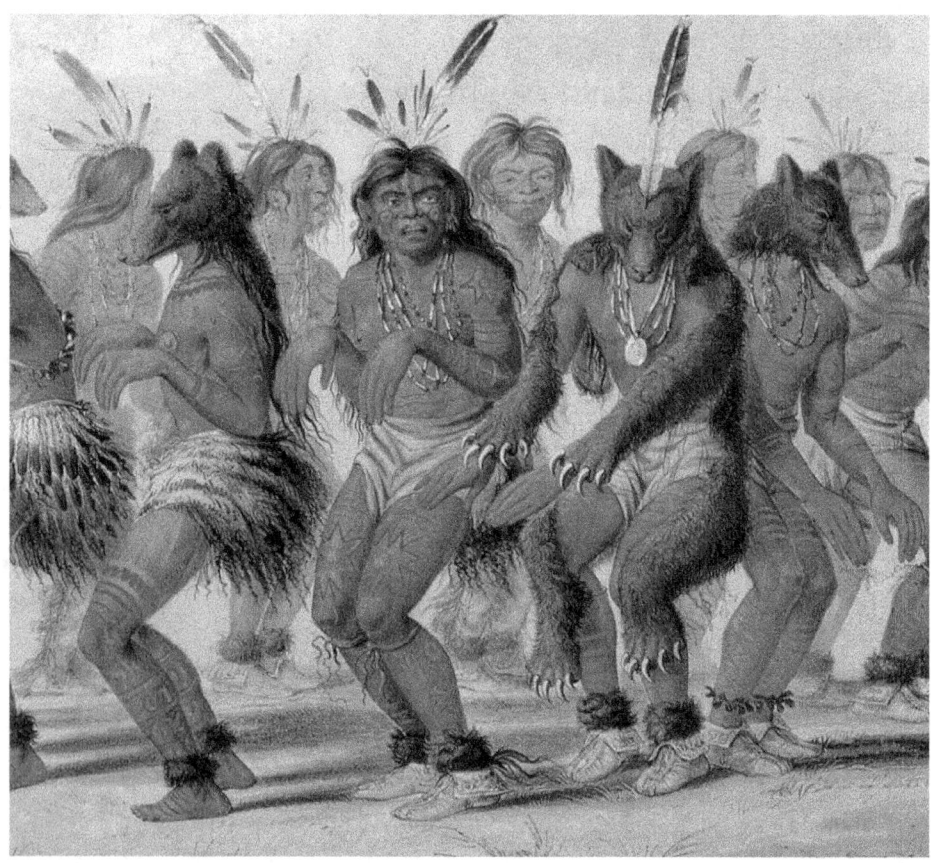

Special structures for healing are often referred to as Medicine Lodges. Wherever they take place, traditional healing ceremonies are considered sacred and are only conducted by Native healers and Native spiritual facilitators. Non-Natives may participate by invitation only.

Indigenous healing practices among Native Americans have been documented in the United States since colonization. Cultural encapsulation has deterred the acknowledgment of Native American medicinal practices as a precursor to folk medicine and many herbal remedies, which have greatly influenced modern medicine.

Understanding Native American healing practices requires helping professionals to know about Native American cultural belief systems about health and wellness, with the many influences that create change in the mind, body, spirit, and natural environment. Native Americans believe their healing practices and traditions operate in the context of relationship to four constructs—namely, spirituality (Creator, Mother Earth, Great Father); community (family, clan, tribe/nation); environment (daily life, nature, balance); and self (inner passions and peace, thoughts, and values).

It is with this in mind, that it's important for today's integrative, complementary medicine practices to become the norm as opposed to the exception. Chief among the ceremonies of Native Americans is the smudging ceremony. Smudging uses the smoking of a variety of herbs and foliage, namely sage and wheatgrass, to be wafted onto the person, belongings, sacred and non-sacred spaces alike. Native Americans differ in their frequency of smudging, but some perform it daily to stay healthy while others only at major life events and when feeling unwell.

While Native American healers' reasonings can vary for why they smudge, from reading many accounts, one of the common reasons is to help others find respect for one another, their environment, and to spend moments in quiet, positive contemplation while practicing this ancient ceremony. In psychology, some of the same tenets of reappraisal and introspection recommended by mental healthcare professionals for greater emotional regulation are given. Here, Native Americans have connected this to their cultural heritage in a way that speaks very meaningfully to the participants

Healing Plants

Native American, Alaska Native, and Native Hawaiian healers all have a long history of using indigenous, or native, plants for a wide variety of medicinal purposes. Medicinal plants and their applications are as diverse as the tribes who use them.

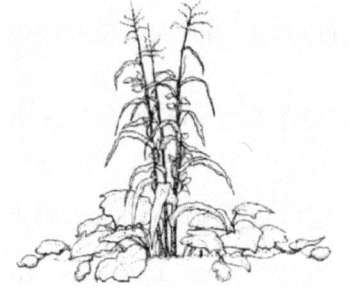

Beyond their medicinal benefits, indigenous plants were a staple of Native people's diet before Western contact. Today, indigenous plants are central to efforts to improve dietary health for current generations. In Hawai'i, the "Waianae Diet" and "Pre-Captain Cook Diet" aim to reduce empty calories, fat, and additives and promote a healthier, more balanced diet by restoring the role of indigenous foods. Alaska Natives and various Indian tribes have similar projects emphasizing traditional foods. Food is medicine.

Native Hawaiian Medicinal Plants

Hawaiian medicinal plants grow in many areas, including in the vicinity of heiaus or temples, sites that are considered sacred. In ancient times, Hawaiian traditional healers would practice La'au Lapa'au, medicinal healing, at some of the heiaus, using plants from around the heiau and in neighboring forests. Most Hawaiian medicinal plants are foods that have additional curative properties. Healers view food as medicine, along with fresh, clean air and water. In all cases, healers offer a prayer to ask permission and give thanks for the medicines before harvesting and preparing them, and ask permission to facilitate medicinal healing on behalf of the Creator

Tools Used In Native American Healing Ceremonies

Well, you are likely to see a modern doctor with a stethoscope hanging on her neck today, the healing implements of the Native American persuasion are equally distinct. Native American healers can be seen with ceremonial headdresses and necklaces of their own making. For healing ceremonies such as those described above, you will find in use a variety of tools from animal totems to peace pipes, prayer ties, and more.

Animal Totems

Since Native American cultures are strongly animistic, animals hold special places in the Native American healing ceremonies and traditions. You can see small animal totems given and used throughout these healing practices, especially during group healing ceremonies, for guidance from their animal spirits.

Dreamcatchers

One of the most iconic Native American healing tools is the dreamcatcher. Representing the Medicine Wheel, or Sacred Hoop, these woven healing instruments are used to help children sleep better, protecting warriors and others traveling away from the tribe, and warding off illness by restoring the balance of mind, emotion, body, and spirit to the person afflicted.

Feather Fetishes

Not what it sounds like, feather fetishes are fans made out of bird feathers, bones, leathered skins of various animals, even seashells, that are used in rituals for prayer and healing. In smudging ceremonies, feather fetishes are used to fan the smoke onto the person being blessed or healed.

Peace Pipes

Peace pipes are a ceremonial tool used usually by elders of a village for major events, but they are also used to smoke a variety of different plants (e.g., peyote, ayahuasca, and other entheogenic herbs). These peace pipes are long-stemmed and typically made of wood or bone, and can be smoked throughout the evening until dawn in healing rituals.

Prayer Ties

Next, prayer ties—small, bound cloth flags—are used as offerings to the Spirit World entities. These colorful little items are laid out to pay homage and thanks to the spirits needed to heal a person.

Smudge Sticks

Finally, but most often used in Native American healing ceremonies, smudge sticks are ribbon-bound herbs used to handily carry and purpose in the smudging ceremonies wherever one might be. Smudge sticks are disassembled to take what herbs are needed for a specific healing ceremony, then the remaining is rebound for later use. Herbs used vary based on the available plant life indigenous to the various Native American nations' regions.

Native American Healing Ceremonies

In addition to the tools mentioned above healers of every Native American tribe extend their toolkit to the knowledge of plant-based medicine. Herbalists didn't simply use smudge sticks to heal afflicted individuals. They had an arsenal of remedies cultivated over generations to handle a variety of ailments that became the source of many modern medicines.

If you would like to gain greater insights into Native American herbalism, in Sacred Plant Medicine: The Wisdom in Native American Herbalism by Stephen Harrod Buhner, he reveals that the Native American cultures not only had spiritual and religious beliefs connected to their herbalism, but an in-depth method for planting, gathering, and harvesting, storing, converting plants to medicine, and uses.

You can find many herbs, such as milkweed, echinacea, wild ginger, and elder in various forms in your local natural foods stores in the supplements section. And, you can thank Native Americans mostly for that!

These herbs are used in many rituals and ceremonies as teas and other concoctions that not only the afflicted person would drink, but many times the family and other members of the tribe, as a means to bond the healing process to the community. Healing is culturally a communal practice and the use of herbs together reinforces that premise.

Death Ceremonies: Native Americans celebrated death, knowing that it was an end to life on Earth, but, believing it to be the start of life in the Spirit World. Most tribes also believed that the journey might be long, so afterlife rituals were performed to ensure that the spirits would not continue to roam the earth. Various tribes honored the dead in several ways, by giving them food, herbs, and gifts to ensure a safe journey to the afterlife.

Green Corn Festivals: Also called the Green Corn Ceremonies, this both a celebration and religious ceremony, primarily practiced by the peoples of the Eastern Woodlands and the Southeastern tribes including the Creek, Cherokee, Seminole, Yuchi, Iroquois, and others. The ceremony typically coincides in the late summer and is tied to the ripening of the corn crops. Marked with dancing, feasting, fasting, and religious observations, the ceremony usually lasts for three days. Activities varied from tribe to tribe, but the common thread is that the corn was not to be eaten until the Great Spirit has been given his proper thanks. During the event, tribal members give thanks for the corn, rain, sun, and a good harvest. Some tribes even believe that they were made from corn by the

Great Spirits. The Green Corn Festival is also a religious renewal, with various religious ceremonies. During this time, some tribes hold council meetings where many of the previous year's minor problems or crimes are forgiven. Others also signify the event as the time of year when youth come of age and babies are given their names. Several tribes incorporate ball games and tournaments in the event. Cleansing and purifying activities often occur, including cleaning out homes, burning waste, and drinking emetics to purify the body. At the end of each day of the festival, feasts are held to celebrate the good harvest. Green Corn festivals are still practiced today by many different native peoples of the Southeastern Woodland Culture.

CHAPTER 2: TRADITIONAL REMEDIES FOR COMMON AILMENTS

Native American Medicine Today

Definition

According to Ken "Bear Hawk" Cohen, "Native American medicine is based on widely held beliefs about healthy living, the repercussions of disease-producing behavior, and the spiritual principles that restore balance." These beliefs are shared by all tribes; however, the methods of diagnosis and treatment vary greatly from tribe to tribe and healer to healer.

Origins

The healing traditions of Native Americans have been practiced in North America since at least 12,000 years ago and possibly as early as 40,000 years ago. Although the term Native American medicine implies that there is a standard system of healing, there are approximately 500 nations of indigenous people in North America, each representing a diverse wealth of healing knowledge, rituals, and ceremonies. Many aspects of

Native American healing have been kept secret and are not written down. The traditions are passed down by word of mouth from elders, from the spirits in vision quests, and through initiation. It is believed that sharing healing knowledge too readily or casually will weaken the spiritual power of the medicine.

There are, however, many Native American healers who recognize that writing down their healing practices is a way to preserve these traditions for future generations. Many also believe that sharing their healing ways and values may help all people to come into a healthier balance with nature and all forms of life.

Benefits

Native American medicine can benefit anyone who sincerely wishes to live a life of wholeness and balance. These benefits may be physical, emotional, or spiritual. There is, however, the understanding that "the diseases of civilization," or white man's diseases, often need white man's medicine. In those cases, Native American medicine can be an important part of an integrative approach to healing. For example, the most successful programs for treating alcohol addiction in Native communities have combined Western approaches to psychological counseling, social work, and traditional Native American healing practices.

Such inherited conditions as birth defects or retardation are not easily treatable with Native American medicine. Native healers also believe that some illnesses are the result of a patient's behavior. Sometimes they will not treat a person because they do not want to interfere with the life lessons the patient needs to learn. Other illnesses are not treated because they are "callings" or initiation diseases.

Description

Native American medicine is based upon a spiritual view of life. A healthy person is someone who has a sense of purpose and follows the guidance of the Great Spirit. This guidance is written upon the heart of every person. To be healthy, a person must be committed to a path of beauty, harmony, and balance. Gratitude, respect, and generosity are also considered to be essential for a healthy life. Ken Cohen writes, "Health means restoring the body, mind, and spirit to balance and wholeness: the balance of life energy in the body; the balance of ethical, reasonable, and just behavior; balanced relations within family and community; and harmonious relationships with nature."

Theories of disease causation and even the names of diseases vary from tribe to tribe. Diseases may be thought to have internal or external causes or sometimes both. According to Cherokee medicine man Rolling Thunder, negative thinking is the most important internal cause of disease. Negative thinking includes not only negative thoughts about oneself but also feelings of shame, blame, low self-esteem, greed, despair, worry, depression, anger, jealousy, and self-centeredness.

Diseases have external causes too. "Germs are also spirits," according to Shabari Bird of the Lakota Nation. A person is particularly susceptible to harmful germs if they live an imbalanced life, have a weak constitution, engage in negative thinking, or are under a lot of stress. Other people or spirits may also be responsible for an illness. Another external source of the disease is environmental poisons. These poisons include alcohol, impure air, water, and some types of food.

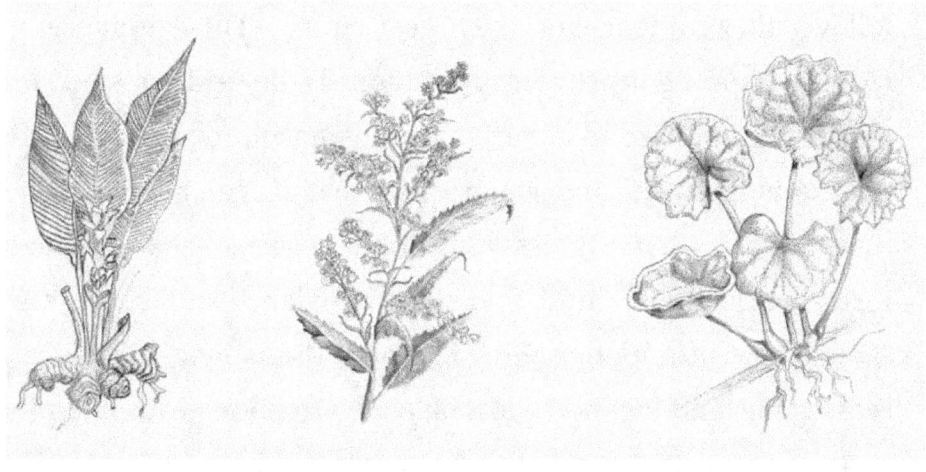

Native American healers believe that disease can also be caused by physical, emotional, or spiritual trauma. These traumas can lead to mental and emotional distress, loss of soul, or loss of spiritual power. In these cases, the healer must use ritual and other ways to physically return the soul and power to the patient. Some diseases are caused when people break the "rules for living." These rules may include ways of showing respect for animals, people, places, ritual objects, events, or spirits.

Native American medicine is not covered by insurance unless perhaps the practitioner is a licensed health care provider. Most Native healers do not charge a set fee for their services. Healing is considered to be "a gift from the Great Spirit." Gifts to the healer are welcomed, however. The offering of a gift "ensures the success of treatment because healing spirits appreciate the generosity." Gifts may include groceries, cloth, money, or another personal expression of respect and appreciation. Frequently the only gift that is required is a pouch of tobacco.

Native Americans used herbs to purify the spirit and bring balance to people who are unhealthy in spirit, mind, or body. They learned about the healing powers of herbs by watching sick animals. Tobacco, one of the most sacred plants to Native Americans, is used in some way in nearly every cure. It is smoked pure and is not mixed with chemicals. Sage, an abundant and pretty plant with blue flowers and light white or grayish leaves, is believed to protect against bad spirits and to draw them out of the body or the soul. Native Americans use sage for many purposes: to heal problems of the stomach, colon, nasal passages, kidneys, liver, lungs, pores of the skin, bones, and sex organs; on the hair and scalp; to heal burns and grazes; as an antiseptic for allergies, colds, and fever; as a gargle for sore throat; and as a tea to calm the nerves. Cedar, a tall evergreen tree, is a milder medicine than sage. It is combined with sage and sweetgrass, a plant that grows in damp environments like marshes or near water, to make a powerful concoction used in the scared smudging ceremony. Cedar fruit and leaves are boiled and then drunk for coughs. Forehead colds, cedar is burned and inhaled.

Traditional Medicine For

Abscess

1. Burdock: Roots and leaves utilized internally and externally. Avoid if pregnant or nursing.

2. Devil's Claw: Used in teas and tonics internally and in poultices externally. Should not be used by women who are or may be pregnant.

3. Chamomile: Commonly used in teas it is best known to help with sleep.

4. Pau d'arco: Long used for a wide range of conditions.

5. Poke: Though parts of this plant are highly toxic to livestock and humans, it has long been used as food and medicine by Native Americans.

6. White Pine: The inner bark, young shoots, twigs, pitch, and leaves have long been used by Native Americans in medical remedies.

7. Slippery Elm: The tree had many traditional uses by Native Americans.

8. Wild Yam: Traditionally used as both food and medicine.

Acne

1. Mint: Dried leaves used in teas and food, found helpful in several remedies.

2. Red Clover: Traditionally used for several conditions.

3. Sarsaparilla: Used for centuries in a wide variety of medicinal remedies.

4. Witch Hazel: Widely used for medicinal purposes by American Indians.

5. Yellow Dock: Native Americans as traditional medicine and food.

6. Buffaloberry: Used as food and in herbal remedies. Overindulgence can cause severe problems including death.

7. Burdock: Roots and leaves utilized internally and externally. Avoid if pregnant or nursing.

Allergies

1. Dong Quai: Used for more than a thousand years to treat several conditions.

2. Mint: Dried leaves used in teas and food, found helpful in several remedies.

3. Rooibos: Used in teas to help with a variety of conditions.

4. Goldenrod: Long used for a variety of ailments.

5. Spirulina: A type of blue-green algae that is rich in protein, vitamins.

Anxiety

1. Kola Nut – Long used in medicinal remedies, spiritual practices, and ceremonies. Should not be used by pregnant or nursing women, or those with intestinal or stomach ulcers, blood pressure, insomnia, or heart disorders.

2. Lavender – Dating back to Roman times, Lavender has been used in teas, balms, food, and medicinal remedies.

3. Lemon Balm – A calming herb that has been used since the Middle Ages.

4. Passion Flower – Has a long history of use among Native Americans that and were adapted by early European colonists. Do not take passionflower if you are pregnant or breastfeeding.

5. Peppermint – in addition to flavoring, long used in traditional medicine for its calming and numbing effects. Should not be used or given to infants or small children.

6. Rhodiola – Best known for improving physical and mental performance.

7. Skullcap – A powerful medicinal herb, it was cultivated by Native Americans for use in several remedies. Pregnant women should not take Skullcap.

8. St John's Wort – Most commonly known as an anti-depressant, it also has other medical uses.

9. Valerian Root – Has been used as a medicinal herb since at least the time of ancient Greece and Rome.

10. Wild Lettuce – Indigenous to North American, it was used for sedative purposes, especially in nervous complaints.

Asthma

1. Damiana – Used internally for a variety of medical issues.

2. Eastern Skunk Cabbage – Dried leaves used as a seasoning in remedies, and as a magical talisman by various tribes.

3. Evening Primrose – Used for both food and medicinal remedies, decoctions were used for internal and external ailments.

4. Feverfew – Used for a variety of internal medical problems. Should not be used by women who are pregnant.

5. Goldenrod – Long used for a variety of ailments.

6. Honeysuckle – Used in traditional herbal remedies for thousands of years.

7. Horehound – Whole plant used internally and externally. People with gastritis or peptic ulcer disorders should use it cautiously.

8. Indian Hemp – A type of marijuana it was used to make clothes, rope, and paper as well as boiling the roots into teas for medicinal problems.

9. Kola Nut – Long used in medicinal remedies, spiritual practices, and ceremonies. Should not be used by pregnant or nursing women, or those with intestinal or stomach ulcers, blood pressure, insomnia, or heart disorders.

10. Lemongrass – Having anti-fungal properties, it has not only been used as herbal medicine but, also as a pesticide and preservative.

11. Mullein – A tobacco-like plant and one of the oldest herbs, it has a long history of use as a medicine

12. Poke – Though parts of this plant are highly toxic to livestock and humans, it has long been used as food and medicine by Native Americans.

13. Rabbit Tobacco – Was thought to have had spiritual or mystic powers by many Indians.

14. Rooibos – Used in teas to help with a variety of conditions.

15. Sumac — Viewed by some tribes as a sacred plant, Sumac was used for both food and medicine.

Backache

1. Arnica — Used externally only for aches, pains, and wounds. Poison if taken internally.

2. Devil's Claw — Used in teas and tonics internally and in poultices externally. Should not be used by a woman who is or may be pregnant. Feverwort — Used internally and externally in herbal medicine.

3. Gentiana — Extremely bitter herb used for both internal and external problems. may irritate persons who have ulcers, and may also cause headaches, nausea, or vomiting.

4. Horsemint — leaves and flowering stems are used in teas, tonics, and salves for a variety of medical issues. Should not be used by pregnant women.

5. Milkweed — Though it can be toxic if not prepared properly, Milkweed was used as a food and medicine, as well as in making cords, ropes, and coarse cloth. Warning: Milkweed may be toxic when taken internally, without sufficient preparation.

Boils

1. Buffaloberry — Used as food and in herbal remedies. Overindulgence can cause severe problems including death.

2. Burdock – Roots and leaves utilized internally and externally. Avoid if pregnant or nursing.

3. Cattail – Utilized as a food, as well as in external and internal medical remedies.

4. Dandelion – Used in both foods and internal and external medical remedies.

5. Devil's Claw – Used in teas and tonics internally and in poultices externally. Should not be used by women who are or may be pregnant.

6. Fenugreek – Used internally and externally for a variety of medicinal purposes.

7. Chamomile – Commonly used in teas it is best known to help with sleep.

8. Greenbriar – Teas and salves used internally and externally.

9. Marshmallow Root – Dating back thousands of years, this root has been used as a food and medicine.

10. Passion Flower – Has a long history of use among Native Americans that and were adapted by early European colonists. Do not take passionflower if you are pregnant or breastfeeding.

11. Prickly Pear Cactus – Native Americans used the younger pads for food and in teas; while mature pads were used in poultices.

12. Pau d'arco – Long used for a wide range of conditions.

13. Slippery Elm – The tree had many traditional uses by Native Americans.

14. Tobacco – Long been important in Native American culture for social, religious, ceremonial purposes as well as in medicinal remedies.

15. White Pine – The inner bark, young shoots, twigs, pitch, and leaves have long been used by Native Americans in medicinal remedies.

16. Wild Yam – Traditionally used as both food and medicine.

Bronchial Infections/Problems

1. Bloodroot – Primarily used as a medicine for respiratory and digestive problems, it also used externally. Today, we know it is toxic and the FDA has classified it as unsafe.

2. Cardinal Flower – Roots, leaf tea, and poultices were used internally and externally.

3. Echinacea – Roots were chewed, dried in tea, or pulverized for external use.

4. Eucalyptus – Teas and ointments used for a variety of purposes.

5. Ginger Root – Utilized as both a spice and medicine throughout the world.

6. Horehound – Whole plant used internally and externally. People with gastritis or peptic ulcer disorders should use it cautiously.

7. Horsemint – leaves and flowering stems are used in teas, tonics, and salves for a variety of medical issues. Should not be used by pregnant women.

8. Kola Nut – Long used in medicinal remedies, spiritual practices, and ceremonies. Should not be used by pregnant or nursing women, or those with intestinal or stomach ulcers, blood pressure, insomnia, or heart disorders.

9. Marshmallow Root – Dating back thousands of years, this root has been used as a food and medicine.

10. Licorice Root – Used as a flavoring in food and for herbal remedies.

11. Plantain – Considered to be one of the nine sacred herbs by the ancient Saxon people and has a long history of use as an alternative medicine dating back to ancient times.

12. Pleurisy Root – Long been found to be effective for many respiratory disorders.

13. Rabbit Tobacco – Was thought to have had spiritual or mystic powers by many Indians.

14. Senna – A large genus of flowering plants found to be helpful in many remedies.

15. Slippery Elm – The tree had many traditional uses by Native Americans.

16. Spearmint – Teas, poultices, and oils used internally and externally for several remedies.

17. Wheat Grass – The result of centuries of cultivation, it is used for numerous medical conditions.

18. White Pine – The inner bark, young shoots, twigs, pitch, and leaves have long been used by Native Americans in medical remedies.

19. Wild Black Cherry – The dried inner bark was traditionally used in tea or syrups for several health problems.

20. Wild Garlic – Used throughout its history for both culinary and medicinal purposes.

Burns

1. Bloodroot – Primarily used as a medicine for respiratory and digestive problems, it also used externally. Today, we know it is toxic and the FDA has classified it as unsafe.

2. Buck Brush – Applies to several North American shrubs used in herbal medicine.

3. Chokecherry – Used as both a source of food and medicine, it was considered one of the most important herbs in Native American medicine.

4. Cattail – Utilized as a food, as well as in external and internal medical remedies.

5. Cotton – Roots, leaves, and seeds have been used in the treatment of many conditions.

6. Greenbriar – Teas and salves used internally and externally.

7. Lavender – Dating back to Roman times, Lavender has been used in teas, balms, food, and medicinal remedies.

8. Mint – Dried leaves used in teas and food, found helpful in several remedies.

9. Oak – Acorns and bark are used for a variety of medical ailments.

10. Pinon – Used so extensively by Native Americans it was referred to by some tribes as the "tree of life."

11. Prickly Pear Cactus – Native Americans used the younger pads for food and in teas; while mature pads were used in poultices.

12. Rabbit Tobacco – Was thought to have had spiritual or mystic powers by many Indians.

13. Sumac – Viewed by some tribes as a sacred plant, Sumac was used for both food and medicine.

14. Western Skunk Cabbage – This plant with a "skunky" has long been used by Native Americans as a topical medicine.

15. Yellow Spined Thistle – Long been used by Native Americans in medicinal remedies.

Cancer

1. Cat's Claw – Used in teas and tonics for more than 2,000 years.

2. Grapefruit – Seeds, pulp, and inner rind used for internal conditions.

3. Green Tea – Made solely with the leaves of Camellia Sinensis, it is known for its many helpful properties.

4. Jiaogulan – Known for its many health-giving qualities and anti-aging effects.

5. Maca – Used for centuries, Maca is consumed as a food and used for medicinal purposes.

6. Oat Straw – A food source and medical remedy since prehistoric times.

7. Olive Oil – A traditional tree crop long used in foods and medicines.

8. Pau d'arco – Long used for a wide range of conditions.

9. Poke – Though parts of this plant are highly toxic to livestock and humans, it has long been used as food and medicine by Native Americans.

10. Rosemary – Used for culinary purposes and in medicinal remedies.

11. Red Clover – Traditionally used for several conditions.

12. Sarsaparilla – Used for centuries in a wide variety of medicinal remedies.

13. Spirulina – A type of blue-green algae that is rich in protein, vitamins.

14. Sumac – Viewed by some tribes as a sacred plant, Sumac was used for both food and medicine.

15. Thistle – This flowering plant of the daisy family, has been used for some 2,000 years for medicinal remedies.

Cough

1. Aspen – Tea was made from the inner bark of the Quaking Aspen tree.

2. American Licorice – Chewed or used in teas for internal issues, in a poultice externally.

3. Black Cohosh – Roots of the plant were used in teas for a variety of ailments.

4. Black Raspberry – Roots and leaves are boiled into tea or chewed, and washes are used externally.

5. Bloodroot – Primarily used as a medicine for respiratory and digestive problems, it also used externally. Today, we know it is toxic and the FDA has classified it as unsafe.

6. Boneset – Dried leaves are used in tea. Caution is advised as it is toxic and has side effects.

7. Broom Snakeweed – Roots and leaves used in steam therapies, teas, and poultices.

8. Chokecherry – Used as both a source of food and medicine, it was considered one of the most important herbs in Native American medicine.

9. Echinacea – Roots were chewed, dried in tea, or pulverized for external use.

10. Eucalyptus – Teas and ointments used for a variety of purposes.

11. Evening Primrose – Used for both food and medicinal remedies, decoctions were used for internal and external ailments.

12. Fennel – Seeds, leaves, and roots used in cooking and medicinal remedies.

13. Gymnema Sylvestre – Has been used as a natural treatment for diabetes for nearly 2,000 years.

14. Hibiscus – Various species used in traditional herbal medicines dating back to Roman times.

15. Horehound – Whole plant used internally and externally. People with gastritis or peptic ulcer disorders should use it cautiously.

16. Horsemint – leaves and flowering stems are used in teas, tonics, and salves for a variety of medical issues. Should not be used by pregnant women.

17. Lemongrass – Having anti-fungal properties, it has not only been used as herbal medicine but, also as a pesticide and preservative.

18. Marshmallow Root – Dating back thousands of years, this root has been used as a food and medicine.

19. Mullein: A tobacco-like plant and one of the oldest herbs, it has a long history of use as a medicine.

20. Osha – Having a wide variety of medicinal properties, Osha was highly valued by Native Americans.

21. Plantain – Considered to be one of the nine sacred herbs by the ancient Saxon people and has a long history of use as an alternative medicine dating back to ancient times.

22. Pleurisy Root – Long been found to be effective for many respiratory disorders.

23. Rabbit Tobacco – Was thought to have had spiritual or mystic powers by many Indians.

24. Rose Hip – The fruit of the rose plant has long been used in teas to soothe a variety of problems.

25. Sage – Used for thousands of years in cooking and like other culinary herbs, it has long been thought to be a digestive aid and appetite stimulant.

26. Saltbush – Many species are used for a variety of conditions.

27. Sarsaparilla – Used for centuries in a wide variety of medicinal remedies.

28. Saw Palmetto – Long prized as a food product, it was also used by Native Americans to make baskets and fans, as well as in medicinal remedies.

29. Schisandra – A genus of a shrub that has many medicinal uses.

30. Senna – A large genus of flowering plants found to be helpful in many remedies.

31. Slippery Elm – The tree had many traditional uses by Native Americans.

32. Star Anise – The fruit of a small tree with a licorice-like flavor long used in medicinal remedies.

33. Sweetflag – Has a very long history of medicinal use in many herbal traditions.

34. Wheat Grass – The result of centuries of cultivation, it is used for numerous medical conditions.

35. White Pine – The inner bark, young shoots, twigs, pitch, and leaves have long been used by Native Americans in medicinal remedies.

Constipation

1. American Ginseng – Used in teas and tonics, it can be an effective laxative.

2. Boneset – Dried leaves are used in tea. Caution is advised as it is toxic and has side effects.

3. Buffaloberry – Used as food and in herbal remedies. Overindulgence can cause severe problems including death.

4. **Cascara Sagrada** – Dried bark used in teas. Bark must be aged and dried thoroughly before use.

5. **Damiana** – Used internally for a variety of medical issues.

6. **Dong Quai** – Used for more than a thousand years to treat several conditions.

7. **Devil's Claw** – Used in teas and tonics internally and in poultices externally. Should not be used by women who are or may be pregnant.

8. **Elder** – Ripe elderberries are used as both food and medicinal remedies.

9. **Fennel** – Seeds, leaves, and roots used in cooking and medicinal remedies.

10. **Fenugreek** – Used internally and externally for a variety of medicinal purposes.

12. **Garcinia Cambogia** – Fruit rind used in a variety of remedies. Not recommended for those with diabetes, people suffering any dementia syndrome, or pregnant and lactating women.

13. **Glucomannan** – A dietary fiber that has long been used in Asia. It is not recommended for use by pregnant or breast-feeding women.

14. Gymnema Sylvestre – Has been used as a natural treatment for diabetes for nearly 2,000 years.

15. Hibiscus – Various species used in traditional herbal medicines dating back to Roman times.

16. Horehound – Whole plant used internally and externally. People with gastritis or peptic ulcer disorders should use it cautiously.

17. Mayapple – Having been long surrounded by folklore, this plant was used for a variety of medical purposes. Because of its toxicity, this herb should only be used by professional Herbalists.

18. Milkweed – Though it can be toxic if not prepared properly, Milkweed was used as a food and medicine, as well as in making cords, ropes, and coarse cloth. **Warning:** Milkweed may be toxic when taken internally, without sufficient preparation.

19. Olive Oil – A traditional tree crop long used in foods and medicines.

20. Persimmon – Long used as food and in traditional medicine.

21. Psyllium Seed Husk – A rich fiber supplement, long used primarily to improve digestion.

22. Senna – A large genus of flowering plants found to be helpful in many remedies.

23. Sumac – Viewed by some tribes as a sacred plant, Sumac was used for both food and medicine.

24. Wheat Grass – The result of centuries of cultivation, it is used for numerous medical conditions.

25. Yellow Dock – Native Americans as traditional medicine and food.

Cramps

1. Blue Cohosh – Root is used in teas and tonics.

2. Cardinal Flower – Roots, leaf tea, and poultices were used internally and externally.

3. Chamomile – Commonly used in teas it is best known to help with sleep.

4. Ginkgo Biloba – One of the most ancient trees in existence, it has been used for both food and medicine.

5. Poke – Though parts of this plant are highly toxic to livestock and humans, it has long been used as food and medicine by Native Americans.

6. St John's Wort – Most commonly known as an anti-depressant, it also has other medical uses.

7. Valerian Root – Has been used as a medicinal herb since at least the time of ancient Greece and Rome.

8. Wild Ginger – Native Americans used the roots as a seasoning as well as a medicinal herb.

Diabetes

1. Allspice – Dried unripe berries have long been used in teas.

2. American Ginseng – Used in teas and tonics, and sometimes smoked by Native Americans.

3. Cat's Claw – Used in teas and tonics for more than 2,000 years.

4. Dandelion – Used in both foods and internal and external medical remedies.

5. Devil's Claw – Used in teas and tonics internally and in poultices externally. Should not be used by a woman who is or may be pregnant.

6. Fenugreek – Used internally and externally for a variety of medicinal purposes.

7. Ginsing – Numerous specifies throughout the world have been used for thousands of years in medical remedies.

8. Goldenrod – Long used for a variety of ailments.

9. Glucomannan – A dietary fiber that has long been used in Asia. It is not recommended for use by pregnant or breast-feeding women.

10. Green Tea – Made solely with the leaves of Camellia Sinensis, it is known for its many helpful properties.

11. Gymnema Sylvestre – Has been used as a natural treatment for diabetes for nearly 2,000 years.

12. Oat Straw – A food source and medical remedy since prehistoric times.

13. Prickly Pear Cactus – Native Americans used the younger pads for food and in teas; while mature pads were used in poultices.

14. Stevia – An herb long used as a sweetener which also has medical remedy properties.

15. Sumac – Viewed by some tribes as a sacred plant, Sumac was used for both food and medicine.

16. Wild Carrot – Used as both food and for health conditions.

17. Yellow Spined Thistle – Long been used by Native Americans in medicinal remedies

Diarrhea

1. American Licorice – Chewed or used in teas for internal issues, in a poultice externally.

2. Blackberry – Tea made from the root-bark is utilized to soothe these types of ailments.

3. Black Raspberry – Roots and leaves are boiled into tea or chewed, and washes are used externally.

4. Boneset – Dried leaves are used in tea. Caution is advised as it is toxic and has side effects.

5. Broom Snakeweed – Roots and leaves used in steam therapies, teas, and poultices.

6. Buckwheat – The fruit seed was used as both a food and in herbal remedies.

7. Cattail – Utilized as a food, as well as in external and internal medical remedies.

8. Cat's Claw – Used in teas and tonics for more than 2,000 years.

9. Chokecherry – Used as both a source of food and medicine, it was considered one of the most important herbs in Native American medicine.

10. Cotton – Roots, leaves, and seeds have been used in the treatment of many conditions.

11. Dandelion – Used in both foods and internal and external medical remedies.

12. Devil's Claw – Used in teas and tonics internally and in poultices externally. Should not be used by women who are or may be pregnant.

13. Dogwood – Bark, berries, and twigs used in decoctions internally and externally.

14. Feverwort – Used internally and externally in herbal medicine.

15. Galangal – Similar to other ginger related herbs, it is primarily used for digestive disorders.

16. Garcinia Cambogia – Fruit rind used in a variety of remedies. Not recommended for those with diabetes, people suffering any dementia syndrome or pregnant and lactating women.

17. Geranium – Scented geranium used in teas for various conditions.

18. Goldenseal – used internally and externally for medicinal issues. Should not be taken by pregnant women.

19. Guarana – Containing caffeine, it has many of the same effects as coffee.

20. Juniper – Used internally and externally for medicinal purposes. Pregnant women should not use this herb as it has been known to cause miscarriage.

21. Marshmallow Root – Dating back thousands of years, this root has been used as a food and medicine.

22. Native Hemlock – Used by Native Americans as a dye, for tanning hides, making baskets and wooden items, as well as medical remedies.

23. Oak – Acorns and bark are used for a variety of medical ailments.

24. Peppermint – In addition to flavoring, long used in traditional medicine for its calming and numbing effects. Should not be used or given to infants or small children.

25. Psyllium Seed Husk – A rich fiber supplement, long used primarily to improve digestion.

26. Rabbit Tobacco – Was thought to have had spiritual or mystic powers by many Indians.

27. Raspberry – Leaves, and fruits used in a wide range of medical issues.

28. Rose Hip – The fruit of the rose plant has long been used in teas to soothe a variety of problems.

29. Sage – Used for thousands of years in cooking and like other culinary herbs, it has long been thought to be a digestive aid and appetite stimulant.

30. Savory – An aromatic herb used as a spice and in folk medicine.

31. Saw Palmetto – Long prized as a food product, it was also used by Native Americans to make baskets and fans, as well as in medical remedies.

32. Sumac – Viewed by some tribes as a sacred plant, Sumac was used for both food and medicine.

33. Uva Ursi – Used medicinally since the second century. Should not be used by pregnant women.

34. Wild Black Cherry – The dried inner bark was traditionally used in tea or syrups for several health problems.

35. Wild Rose – There are hundreds of species that have been used medicinally for thousands of years.

36. Wild Garlic – Used throughout its history for both culinary and medicinal purposes.

37. Willow – The leaves and bark of the willow tree have been used since the times of ancient Egypt and Greece.

Dropsy

1. Blue Cohosh – Root is used in teas and tonics.

2. Eastern Skunk Cabbage – Dried leaves used as a seasoning, in remedies, and as a magical talisman by various tribes.

3. Greenbriar – Teas and salves used internally and externally.

4. Indian Hemp – A type of marijuana it was used to make clothes, rope, and paper as well as boiling the roots into teas for medicinal problems.

5. Milkweed – Though it can be toxic if not prepared properly, Milkweed was used as a food and medicine, as well as in making cords, ropes, and coarse cloth. **Warning:** Milkweed may be toxic when taken internally, without sufficient preparation.

6. Sweetflag – Has a very long history of medicinal use in many herbal traditions.

7. Tobacco – Long been important in Native American culture for social, religious, ceremonial purposes as well as in medicinal remedies.

8. Wild Carrot – Used as both food and for health conditions.

9. Wild Lettuce – Indigenous to North American, it was used for sedative purposes, especially in nervous complaints.

Eye Problems, Irritation, Soreness

1. Black Gum – Used by Native Americans in baths, washes, and tonics.

2. Dandelion – Used in both foods and internal and external medicinal remedies.

3. Fendler's Bladderpod – Used crushed leaves for internal and external use.

4. Fennel – Seeds, leaves, and roots used in cooking and medicinal remedies.

5. Goldenseal – used internally and externally for medicinal issues. Should not be taken by pregnant women.

6. Pennyroyal – Long used to treat medical problems and to eradicate pests. Pennyroyal should not be used in any way by pregnant women. Over ingestion of this herb has caused death.

7. Plantain – Considered to be one of the nine sacred herbs by the ancient Saxon people and has a long history of use as an alternative medicine dating back to ancient times.

8. Sumac – Viewed by some tribes as a sacred plant, Sumac was used for both food and medicine.

9. Wild Black Cherry – The dried inner bark was traditionally used in tea or syrups for several health problems.

10. White Willow – The use of willow bark dates back thousands of years.

Fever

1. American Ginseng – Used in teas and tonics, and sometimes smoked by Native Americans.

2. American Licorice – Chewed or used in teas for internal issues, in a poultice externally.

3. Boswellia – Fragrant resin utilized in a variety of ailments. Should not be used by pregnant, breastfeeding women and children.

4. Broom Snakeweed – Roots and leaves used in steam therapies, teas, and poultices.

5. Buffaloberry – Used as food and in herbal remedies. Overindulgence can cause severe problems including death.

6. Devil's Claw – Used in teas and tonics internally and in poultices externally. Should not be used by women who are or may be pregnant.

7. Dogwood – bark, berries, and twigs used in decoctions internally and externally.

8. Catnip – Stems and leaves make an aromatic tea which is useful for many conditions.

9. Cardinal Flower – Roots, leaf tea, and poultices were used internally and externally.

10. Dandelion – Used in both foods and internal and external medical remedies.

11. Eucalyptus – Teas and ointments used for a variety of purposes.

12. Feverfew – Used for a variety of internal medical problems. Should not be used by women who are pregnant.

13. Feverwort – Used internally and externally in herbal medicine.

14. Ginger Root – Utilized as both a spice and medicine throughout the world.

15. Gymnema Sylvestre – Has been used as a natural treatment for diabetes for nearly 2,000 years.

16. Hibiscus – Various species used in traditional herbal medicines dating back to Roman times.

17. Honeysuckle – Used in traditional herbal remedies for thousands of years.

18. Horsemint – leaves and flowering stems are used in teas, tonics, and salves for a variety of medical issues. Should not be used by pregnant women.

19. Indian Hemp – A type of marijuana it was used to make clothes, rope, and paper as well as boiling the roots into teas for medicinal problems.

20. Native Hemlock – Used by Native Americans as a dye, for tanning hides, making baskets and wooden items, as well as medicinal remedies.

21. Osha – Having a wide variety of medicinal properties, Osha was highly valued by Native Americans.

22. Pau d'arco – Long used for a wide range of conditions.

23. Pennyroyal – Long used to treat medical problems and to eradicate pests. Pennyroyal should not be used in any way by pregnant women. Over ingestion of this herb has caused death.

24. Persimmon – Long used as food and in traditional medicine.

25. Rabbit Tobacco – Was thought to have had spiritual or mystic powers by many Indians.

26. Sarsaparilla – Used for centuries in a wide variety of medicinal remedies.

27. Sassafras – Used extensively for food and medicine by Native Americans long before European settlers arrived.

28. Spearmint – Teas, poultices, and oils used internally and externally for several remedies.

29. Sumac – Viewed by some tribes as a sacred plant, Sumac was used for both food and medicine.

30. Tobacco – Long been important in Native American culture for social, religious, ceremonial purposes as well as in medical remedies.

31. Wild Rose – There are hundreds of species that have been used medicinally for thousands of years.

32. Wheat Grass – The result of centuries of cultivation, it is used for numerous medical conditions.

33. White Pine – The inner bark, young shoots, twigs, pitch, and leaves have long been used by Native Americans in medical remedies.

34. Wild Black Cherry – The dried inner bark was traditionally used in tea or syrups for several health problems.

35. White Willow – The use of willow bark dates back thousands of years.

Flu

1. American Ginseng – Used in teas and tonics, and sometimes smoked by Native Americans.

2. Boneset – Dried leaves are used in tea. Caution is advised as it is toxic and has side effects.

3. Catnip – Stems and leaves make an aromatic tea which is useful for many conditions.

4. Chamomile – Commonly used in teas it is best known to help with sleep.

5. Echinacea – Roots were chewed, dried in tea, or pulverized for external use.

6. Elder – Ripe elderberries are used as both a food and in medicinal remedies.

7. Eleuthero – Dried roots have been used for centuries. People with medicated high blood pressure should consult their doctor, can cause insomnia.

8. Feverwort – Used internally and externally in herbal medicine.

9. Ginger Root – Utilized as both a spice and medicine throughout the world.

10. Goldenrod – Long used for a variety of ailments.

11. Goldenseal – used internally and externally for medicinal issues. Should not be taken by pregnant women.

12. Green Tea – Made solely with the leaves of Camellia Sinensis, it is known for its many helpful properties.

13. Mint – Dried leaves used in teas and food, found helpful in several remedies.

14. Native Hemlock – Used by Native Americans as a dye, for tanning hides, making baskets and wooden items, as well as medicinal remedies.

15. Osha – Having a wide variety of medicinal properties, Osha was highly valued by Native Americans.

16. Pau d'arco – Long used for a wide range of conditions.

17. Pleurisy Root – Long been found to be effective for many respiratory disorders.

18. Rabbit Tobacco – Was thought to have had spiritual or mystic powers by many Indians.

19. Sage – Used for thousands of years in cooking and like other culinary herbs, it has long been thought to be a digestive aid and appetite stimulant.

20. Sassafras – Used extensively for food and medicine by Native Americans long before European settlers arrived.

21. Star Anise – The fruit of a small tree with a licorice-like flavor long used in medicinal remedies.

22. White Pine – The inner bark, young shoots, twigs, pitch, and leaves have long been used by Native Americans in medicinal remedies.

23. Wild Black Cherry – The dried inner bark was traditionally used in tea or syrups for several health problems.

Heartburn

1. Dandelion – Used in both foods and internal and external medical remedies.

2. Ginger Root – Utilized as both a spice and medicine throughout the world.

3. Licorice Root – Used as a flavoring in food and for herbal remedies.

4. Mint – Dried leaves used in teas and food, found helpful in several remedies.

5. Osha – Having a wide variety of medicinal properties, Osha was highly valued by Native Americans.

6. Peppermint – In addition to flavoring, long used in traditional medicine for its calming and numbing effects. Should not be used or given to infants or small children.

7. Rooibos – Used in teas to help with a variety of conditions.

8. Stevia – An herb long used as a sweetener which also has medical remedy properties.

9. White Pine – The inner bark, young shoots, twigs, pitch, and leaves have long been used by Native Americans in medical remedies.

10. Wormwood – The leaves and flowering tops were gathered and dried to use in medicinal tonics.

Infection

1. Cattail – Utilized as a food, as well as in external and internal medical remedies.

2. Echinacea – Roots were chewed, dried in tea, or pulverized for external use.

3. Eucalyptus – Teas and ointments used for a variety of purposes.

4. Grapefruit – Seeds, pulp, and inner rind used for internal conditions.

5. Goldenseal – used internally and externally for medicinal issues. Should not be taken by pregnant women.

6. Spirulina – A type of blue-green algae that is rich in protein, vitamins.

7. Wild Rose – There are hundreds of species that have been used medicinally for thousands of years.

8. Wheat Grass – The result of centuries of cultivation, it is used for numerous medical conditions.

Inflammation/Swelling

1. American Ginseng – Used in teas and tonics, and sometimes smoked by Native Americans.

2. American Licorice – Chewed or used in teas for internal issues, in a poultice externally.

3. Arnica – Used externally only for aches, pains, and wounds. Poison if taken internally.

4. Ashwagandha – The whole plant is used in numerous remedies. Caution is advised in the use of this plant since it is toxic.

5. Blackberry – Tea made from the root-bark is utilized to soothe these types of ailments.

6. Boswellia – Fragrant resin utilized in a variety of ailments. Should not be used by pregnant, breastfeeding women and children.

7. Buck Brush – Applies to several North American shrubs used in herbal medicine.

8. Buffaloberry – Used as food and in herbal remedies. Overindulgence can cause severe problems including death.

9. Cat's Claw – Used in teas and tonics for more than 2,000 years.

10. Cattail – Utilized as a food, as well as in external and internal medical remedies.

11. Chasteberry – Berries and flowers used in teas. Pregnant or breast-feeding women should not take a chaste berry.

12. Dandelion – Used in both foods and internal and external medical remedies.

13. Devil's Claw – Used in teas and tonics internally and in poultices externally. Should not be used by women who are or may be pregnant.

14. Echinacea – Roots were chewed, dried in tea, or pulverized for external use.

15. Elder – Ripe elderberries are used as both a food and in medicinal remedies.

16. Eleuthero – Dried roots have been used for centuries. People with medicated high blood pressure should consult their doctor, can cause insomnia.

17. Eucalyptus – Teas and ointments used for a variety of purposes.

18. Evening Primrose – Used for both food and medicinal remedies, decoctions were used for internal and external ailments.

19. Fenugreek – Used internally and externally for a variety of medicinal purposes.

20. Garcinia Cambogia – Fruit rind used in a variety of remedies. Not recommended for those with diabetes, people suffering any dementia syndrome or pregnant and lactating women.

21. Gentiana – Extremely bitter herb used for both internal and external problems. May irritate persons who have ulcers, and may also cause headache, nausea, or vomiting.

22. Green Tea – Made solely with the leaves of Camellia Sinensis, it is known for its many helpful properties.

23. Horsemint – leaves and flowering stems are used in teas, tonics, and salves for a variety of medical issues. Should not be used by pregnant women.

24. Lavender – Dating back to Roman times, Lavender has been used in teas, balms, food, and medicinal remedies.

25. Marshmallow Root – Dating back thousands of years, this root has been used as a food and medicine.

26. Mullein – A tobacco-like plant and one of the oldest herbs, it has a long history of use as a medicine.

27. Oak – Acorns and bark are used for a variety of medical ailments.

28. Pleurisy Root – Long been found to be effective for many respiratory disorders.

29. Poke – Though parts of this plant are highly toxic to livestock and humans, it has long been used as food and medicine by Native Americans.

30. Raspberry – Leaves, and fruits used in a wide range of medical issues.

31. Rose Hip – The fruit of the rose plant has long been used in teas to soothe a variety of problems.

32. Skullcap – A powerful medicinal herb, it was cultivated by Native Americans for use in several remedies. Pregnant women should not take Skullcap.

33. St John's Wort – Most commonly known as an anti-depressant, it also has other medical uses.

34. Sweetflag – Has a very long history of medicinal use in many herbal traditions.

35. Western Skunk Cabbage – This plant with a "skunky" has long been used by Native Americans as a topical medicine.

36. Wild Rose – There are hundreds of species that have been used medicinally for thousands of years.

37. White Pine – The inner bark, young shoots, twigs, pitch, and leaves have long been used by Native Americans in medical remedies

38. Wild Black Cherry – The dried inner bark was traditionally used in tea or syrups for several health problems.

39. White Willow – The use of willow bark dates back thousands of years.

40. Witch Hazel – Widely used for medicinal purposes by American Indians.

Insect Bites And Stings

1. Bloodroot – Primarily used as a medicine for respiratory and digestive problems, it also used externally. Today, we know it is toxic and the FDA has classified it as unsafe.

2. Broom Snakeweed – Roots and leaves used in steam therapies, teas, and poultices.

3. Buffaloberry – Used as food and in herbal remedies. Overindulgence can cause severe problems including death.

4. Goldenseal – used internally and externally for medicinal issues. Should not be taken by pregnant women.

5. Honeysuckle – Used in traditional herbal remedies for thousands of years.

6. Lavender – Dating back to Roman times, Lavender has been used in teas, balms, food, and medicinal remedies.

7. Lemon Balm – A calming herb that has been used since the Middle Ages.

8. Osha – Having a wide variety of medicinal properties, Osha was highly valued by Native Americans.

9. Plantain – Considered to be one of the nine sacred herbs by the ancient Saxon people and has a long history of use as an alternative medicine dating back to ancient times.

10. Saltbush – Many species are used for a variety of conditions.

11. Stiff Goldenrod – Long been used to stop bleeding and other ailments.

Menstrual Cramps And Pain

1. Allspice – Dried unripe berries have long been used in teas.

2. Black Cohosh – Roots of the plant were used in teas for a variety of ailments.

3. Dong Quai – Used for more than a thousand years to treat several conditions.

4. Ginger Root – Utilized as both a spice and medicine throughout the world.

5. Hibiscus – Various species used in traditional herbal medicines dating back to Roman times.

6. Horehound – Whole plant used internally and externally. People with gastritis or peptic ulcer disorders should use it cautiously.

7. Osha – Having a wide variety of medicinal properties, Osha was highly valued by Native Americans.

8. Partridgeberry – Used as food and medical problems, primarily for women.

9. Peppermint – in addition to flavoring, long used in traditional medicine for its calming and numbing effects. Should not be used or given to infants or small children.

10. Sage – Used for thousands of years in cooking and like other culinary herbs, it has long been thought to be a digestive aid and appetite stimulant.

11. Spearmint – Teas, poultices, and oils used internally and externally for several remedies.

12. Wild Yam – Traditionally used as both food and medicine.

Pneumonia

1. Dogwood – Bark, berries, and twigs used in decoctions internally and externally.

2. Honeysuckle – Used in traditional herbal remedies for thousands of years.

3. Pleurisy Root – Long been found to be effective for many respiratory disorders.

4. Rabbit Tobacco – Was thought to have had spiritual or mystic powers by many Indians.

5. White Pine – The inner bark, young shoots, twigs, pitch, and leaves have long been used by Native Americans in medical remedies.

6. Wild Black Cherry – The dried inner bark was traditionally used in tea or syrups for several health problems.

Stomach Problems

1. Allspice – Dried unripe berries have long been used in teas.

2. American Licorice – Chewed or used in teas for internal issues, in a poultice externally.

3. Blackberry – Root is used in teas, and leaves are used as a gargle.

4. Black Raspberry – Roots and leaves are boiled into tea or chewed, and washes are used externally.

5. Boswellia – Fragrant resin utilized in a variety of ailments. Should not be used by pregnant, breast-feeding women and children.

6. Dandelion – Used in both foods and internal and external medicinal remedies.

7. Devil's Claw – Used in teas and tonics internally and in poultices externally. Should not be used by a woman who is or may be pregnant.

8. Fennel – Seeds, leaves, and roots used in cooking and medicinal remedies.

9. Fenugreek – Used internally and externally for a variety of medicinal purposes.

10. Feverfew – Used for a variety of internal medical problems. Should not be used by women who are pregnant.

11. Ginger Root – Utilized as both a spice and medicine throughout the world.

12. Grapefruit – Seeds, pulp, and inner rind used for internal conditions.

13. Greenbriar – Teas and salves used internally and externally.

14. Pennyroyal – Long used to treat medical problems and to eradicate pests. Pennyroyal should not be used in any way by pregnant women. Over ingestion of this herb has caused death.

15. Peppermint – In addition to flavoring, long used in traditional medicine for its calming and numbing effects. Should not be used or given to infants or small children.

Syphilis

1. Boswellia – Fragrant resin utilized in a variety of ailments. Should not be used by pregnant, breast-feeding women and children.

2. Cardinal Flower – Roots, leaf tea, and poultices were used internally and externally.

3. Geranium – Scented geranium used in teas for various conditions.

4. Pinon – Used so extensively by Native Americans it was referred to by some tribes as the "tree of life."

5. Poke – Though parts of this plant are highly toxic to livestock and humans, it has long been used as food and medicine by Native Americans.

6. Sarsaparilla – Used for centuries in a wide variety of medicinal remedies.

7. Yellow Spined Thistle – Long been used by Native Americans in medicinal remedies.

Wounds

1. Arnica – Used externally only for aches, pains, and wounds. Poison if taken internally.

2. Broom Snakeweed – Roots and leaves used in steam therapies, teas, and poultices.

3. Buck Brush – Applies to several North American shrubs used in herbal medicine.

4. Buffaloberry – Used as food and in herbal remedies

5. Cattail – Utilized as a food, as well as in external and internal medical remedies.

6. Chokecherry – Used as both a source of food and medicine, it was considered one of the most important herbs in Native American medicine.

7. Cotton – Roots, leaves, and seeds have been used in the treatment of many conditions.

8. Dogwood – Bark, berries, and twigs used in decoctions internally and externally.

9. Echinacea – Roots were chewed, dried in tea, or pulverized for external use.

10. Eucalyptus – Teas and ointments used for a variety of purposes.

11. Evening Primrose – Used for both food and medicinal remedies, decoctions were used for internal and external ailments.

12. Fenugreek – Used internally and externally for a variety of medicinal purposes.

13. Gentiana – Extremely bitter herb used for both internal and external problems. May irritate persons who have ulcers, and may also cause headache, nausea.

14. Goldenrod – Long used for a variety of ailments.

15. Goldenseal – Used internally and externally for medicinal issues. Should not be taken by pregnant women.

CHAPTER 3: MOST COMMON DIY HERBAL RECIPES

1. Tea

1. Lemon And Elderflower Tea For Fighting Common Flu

Elderflowers and lemon might easily become your most favorite herbal tea in the world. While lemon tea is no stranger to tea drinkers, elderflowers are still not as widely used as they deserve. Some studies showed that elderberry flowers may have help to relieve flu symptoms. However, the best part of elderflower tea is – the flavor. Because of their unique and sweet flavor, these flowers are popular for making syrups and flavoring soft drinks and water. They blend amazingly well with lemon too. You can use both fresh and dry flowers. Wash them before use. Elderflower usually grows freely in nature and start blooming around May.

Blend: (For 1 Cup)

- ❖ 1 spoon of elderflowers
- ❖ 1-2 teaspoons of lemon juice
- ❖ 1 teaspoon of honey

2. Ginger Tea

Fresh, dried, pickled, or powdered, ginger tastes well in any form and in any dish or drink – especially in tea. Ginger tea is the only tea we recommend making with fresh instead of dry ingredients. Peel, wash, and slice ginger into thin slices. Then add it to a small saucepan together with 1 ½ cup of water and a few peppercorns. Bring it to a boil and let it simmer for another 10-15 minutes. Strain, add honey, and drink. Why adding peppercorns to a blend? Both ginger and peppercorns may warm you up, may offer benefits for the digestive system, and positively influence the mood.

Blend: (For One Cup)

- ❖ ½ – 1 inch of fresh ginger
- ❖ A teaspoon of honey
- ❖ A few peppercorns

3. Mint And Lavender

Upgrade the simple mint tea by adding a touch of lavender flowers. Lavender may help with relaxation, and help freshen the breath. Together with mint, it gives a delicious and potent tea with relaxing, antimicrobial, antiviral, and antioxidant properties. To brew mint and lavender tea, use about 1 teaspoon of dry leaves. Bring water to a boil and let it cool for a few minutes. Oversteeped lavender tea may become bitter. You can easily fix this by adding a spoon of honey. Once brewed, you can cool it down and serve it with honey and ice as iced tea.

Blend: (For 2 Cups)

- ❖ 1 spoon of mint
- ❖ ¼ spoon of lavender flowers
- ❖ 1 teaspoon of honey

4. Herbal Chai Tea

Nothing beats a cup of warm chai – in any season. While the real chai is made with strong black tea, herbal chai has no caffeine at all. This warm and soothing drink can be made with powdered or crushed spices. The best base for herbal chai is pure rooibos tea. It's strong enough to hold all the spices and blends well with milk. Rooibos is naturally lightly sweet, and won't have a bitter taste even if over-brewed.

Blend: (For 4-5 Cups)

- ❖ 4 spoons of rooibos tea
- ❖ 1 teaspoon of ginger powder
- ❖ 2 inches of crushed cinnamon bark
- ❖ ½ -1 teaspoon of crushed cardamom

- ½ -1 teaspoon of cloves

2. Decoctions

What Is An Herbal Decoction?

So, what precisely is an herbal decoction? A decoction is an herbal preparation created by boiling herbs in liquid, usually water. Herbalist James Green explains, "the object of preparing decoctions is to secure, in aqueous solution, the soluble active principles of herbs that are hard and woody and have a close, dense texture"

1. Roasted Dandelion Root Tea Recipe

Ingredients

- 4½ tsp dried dandelion root (where to buy dandelion root if you can't find it locally)
- 2 cups of water
- 1 to 2 tbsp butter or cream to taste (optional)
- Optional additions - 1 cinnamon stick OR 1/2 teaspoon of dried ginger OR 1 teaspoon fresh minced ginger. OR vanilla extract to taste (or a combination of these)

Instructions

- Place a medium pot over medium heat and place the dried dandelion root in the bottom.

- Toast the root until it becomes fragrant and golden brown, then add water and additional flavorings (if using) and bring to a boil.
- When the water boils, reduce heat and allow to simmer for 30-45 minutes, then strain and serve.
- Blend in a little maple syrup and a tablespoon of butter, or try a dollop of cream and 2-3 drops of vanilla extract.

Marshmallow Decoction Recipe

- 1.5 cups water
- 1 tablespoon cut and sifted marshmallow root

Instructions: Bring water and marshmallow to a boil, then cover and simmer on low for 20 minutes. Remove from heat, strain with a mesh strainer or cheesecloth, and sweeten if desired before serving.

3. Popsicles

Popsicles Made With Chamomile And Hibiscus

Ingredients

- 2 tablespoons dry chamomile
- 1 tablespoon dry hibiscus
- 1 ¼ cups boiling water
- 1 cup greek yogurt
- Honey to taste

- Pinch of salt
- 1 tablespoon lemon juice
- Popsicle molds (you can use paper cups and Popsicle sticks)

Instructions

- Begin your Popsicles by making a tea out of the chamomile and hibiscus. Put the herbs in a cup, pour water over the herbs, and let steep for five minutes. (sometimes waiting is the hardest part)
- Strain into a small bowl
- While the mixture is still hot, add honey to taste. Stir well so the honey combines well with the tea. You will be mixing this with the yogurt so you may want to make it more on the sweet side.
- Add a pinch of salt
- Add the lemon juice. You can use the juice of fresh lemon. We keep this type of fresh lemon juice on hand for convenience.
- Let the mixture cool a little
- Add the yogurt and mix well
- Pour into the Popsicle molds
- Places these in the freezer until frozen solid

Lavender Plus Lemon Balm Popsicles

Ingredients

- 4 cups of water
- 5-6 whole fresh lavender blossoms
- 1 small handful of fresh lemon balm
- 2-4 tbsp honey

Instructions

- Bring the water to a boil, then pour over the lavender and lemon balm in a quart-sized jar.
- Steep the tea for 10-15 minutes, then strain out the herbs with a fine-mesh sieve and stir in the honey to your desired sweetness.
- Let the tea cool down a bit (you can add a few ice cubes if you're impatient like me), then pour it into a popsicle mold. Freeze for several hours or overnight.

Sunshine Pops

Ingredients:

- 2 tablespoons chamomile
- 2 tablespoons lemon balm
- 2 tablespoons milky oats (or oatstraw)
- 1 teaspoon lavender
- Peel from ¼ of a lemon
- Honey to taste

- Bee pollen to taste (optional)

Directions:

- Prepare your tea or infusion by pouring 4 cups of boiling water over the herbs and lemon peel.
- Steep for 30 min and taste. If you would like a stronger brew, steep for an additional 30 minutes and then strain. Mix in honey to taste.
- Pour liquid into your popsicle mold of choice and freeze for one hour.
- After one hour, add in the bee pollen to the molds and gently combine and then insert popsicle sticks into each pop and freeze for an additional four hours, or until completely frozen

4. Ice Cubes

Ingredients

- Herbs, of choice (basil, chives, cilantro, fennel, lovage, mint, oregano, parsley, rosemary, sage, tarragon, thyme)
- Boiling water

Directions

- Mince herb (s) of choice.
- Pack minced herb (s) into an ice cube tray, each 3/4 full.

- Fill with boiling water, (this will blanch the herbs before freezing and will help them retain their flavor and color).
- Once the herbal ice cubes are frozen, you can pop them out of their tray and into freezer bags for storage.
- Use as needed.

Herb Infused Ice Cubes

Ingredients

- Ice Cube Tray
- Fresh herbs
- Water

Directions

- Fill each section of an ice cube tray with fresh herbs.
- Fill the ice cube tray with boiling water. This will blanch the herbs and help them retain their color and flavor.
- Freeze

5. Bath

Spring Tea Bath

Materials:

- Five 5" x 7" sized muslin bags or cheesecloth
- Big mixing bowl
- Spoon for mixing
- Cooking twine or cotton string (if using cheesecloth)

Ingredients

- 1 cup dried lavender flowers
- 1 cup dried rose petals
- 1 cup dried chamomile flowers
- 1 cup dried calendula petals
- 1 cup dried red clover blossoms

Instructions

- Pour flowers into a mixing bowl and blend them.
- Fill each muslin bag with the flour mixture or use cheesecloth and twine to create a small pouch.
- Tie shut and use one bag per bath. The bag can be tied to the water spout for the hot water to run through, or simply placed in the tub to float like a teabag in an infusion.

6. Breast milk

1. Fennel Seeds

Fennel seeds are great for increasing the milk supply in nursing mothers. It has phytoestrogens, similar to estrogen, which is a hormone that also helps in producing more milk

Instructions

- You can use fennel seeds to make tea by infusing them in hot water for a few minutes. You can add honey for sweetness (optional). You may take this tea a couple of times a day. If you are not very enthusiastic about tea, you may chew a spoonful of Add- roasted seeds a few times a day.

2. Torbagun Leaves

This is a great herb for breastfeeding. Torbagun leaves are popularly used in Bataknese cuisine, but they have been in use for centuries for improving lactation in breastfeeding mothers.

Instructions

- ❖ You may use these miraculous leaves in any form. You may take half a teaspoon or so of the leaves and add them to a cup of boiling water to make some tea, add it to your soup, or your regular vegetable preparation and consume it regularly.

3. Fenugreek Seeds

Fenugreek seeds are one of the best herbs for breastfeeding mothers to increase milk production. It also contains diosgenin and phytoestrogen. These seeds are also loaded with galactagogue, which makes them great for mothers who wish to enhance their breast milk supply

How To Use

- ❖ You may take a teaspoon full of fenugreek seeds and boil them in water. Strain the seeds. You may add a teaspoonful of honey and a pinch of turmeric to this to enhance the taste. Drink this tea at least two to three times a day. Mix fenugreek sprouts with salad or veggies as well.

4. Shatavari

This Ayurvedic herb has been in use to overcome lactation problems in women. This herb has galactagogue properties that help increase the production of prolactin and corticoids, which help produce breast milk, which in turn improve lactation and the quality of breast milk too

How To Use

- ❖ You may take this herb by mixing it in water, or you may also buy Shatavari herbal supplements for increasing breast milk supply.

5. Cinnamon

Cinnamon is a fragrant herb that enriches the flavors of many culinary dishes. However, for a long time, many breastfeeding mothers who suffer from insufficient milk supply have been using this herb to increase their milk flow. It is also said to enhance the flavor of breast milk.

How To Use

- ❖ Lactating mothers may consume cinnamon by mixing a pinch of cinnamon powder in warm water, half a teaspoon of honey, or by adding it to milk. You may take cinnamon for a month or two to see the difference in your breast milk supply.

6. Anise

This herb has estrogenic properties; it contains anethole, which is a phytoestrogen. which helps unblocked clogged milk ducts and increases breast milk supply

How To Use

- ❖ You may make tea by infusing a few anise seeds in hot water. Add sugar or honey for taste. You may safely consume two to three cups in a day.

- ❖ The availability of these ayurvedic/natural herbs may make you pick some of them and begin consuming them right away. However, it's not as simple because you must consume what is healthy for your baby. Additionally, your body may not react the way it used to before after consuming the same ingredients. But you need not worry. Take these precautionary measures to ensure you gain the most health benefits from these ayurvedic herbs

7. Compresses

Cold Herbal Compresses

Materials:

- 2-4 cotton or linen washcloths
- Large glass bowl
- Plate/ lid for the glass bowl

Ingredients:

- Two herbal tea bags per each towel.
- Tea suggestions: Chamomile-Lavender, Green Tea Peppermint, and Peppermint.
- 1 cup of water per each towel used
- Essential oil suggestions:
- Lavender: calming and soothing
- Peppermint: energizing and cooling
- Eucalyptus: invigorating and awakening

Directions:

- **Make A Tea Concentrate:** Bring water to a boil. Place tea bags in a glass bowl, and cover with water. Cover and let steep for 15-20 minutes, until thoroughly cooled or place in the refrigerator to chill quickly.
- Soak a clean cotton or linen washcloth in the tea concentrate and allow it to become fully saturated. Then gently squeeze any excess tea out of the cloth. It should be heavy and wet, but not dripping.

- Lay towel flat, and apply two drops of desired essential oil. Be careful – we don't recommend applying undiluted essential oil directly onto your skin.
- Roll or fold the washcloth and apply it to the head, neck, chest, or feet.
- Relax and enjoy this restorative herbal practice.

8. Poultice

Ingredients

- 2-3 tablespoons (or more as needed) of fresh or dried herbs, healing clays, or activated charcoal as needed
- Enough hot water to form a thick paste
- Organic cheesecloth or cloth for covering
- Waterproof covering to keep poultice on

Instructions

- Make a thick paste with the desired herb, clay or charcoal, and water.
- Apply directly to the wound or place between two layers of cloth and apply the cloth to the wound (depending on the cloth and the wound). Leave for 20 minutes to 3 hours as needed and repeat as necessary.

Making A Soothing Yarrow Poultice

You Will Need:

- 25-50 g fresh yarrow herb (a good handful of the leaf)
- Water
- Pestle and mortar, muslin and scissors
- Pick leaves and brush off insects and dirt.
- Chop or tear the herb coarsely, and place in the mortar.
- Add a little water and crush and mash herbs into pulp or paste using the pestle.
- Cut a piece of muslin about twice the area of skin to be treated, and spread the herb paste onto the layer of muslin. Fold over the muslin onto the herb, like a sandwich.
- Apply the muslin with herb paste direct to the affected area, tie on with strips of muslin, leave on for 30 min, and repeat as needed.

What You'll Need:

- 1 teaspoon turmeric powder
- 1 ounce freshly chopped or grated ginger
- ¼ small raw sliced onion
- 1 chopped garlic clove
- 2 teaspoons coconut oil
- cheesecloth or cotton bandage

How To Do It:

- Add the coconut oil followed by the rest of the ingredients to a pan on low heat and allow it to heat until it's almost dry but not burnt.
- Turn off the stove and transfer ingredients to a bowl to cool so that it's warm to the touch.
- Lay the cloth flat and add the mixture to the center of the cloth.
- Fold the cloth over twice to create a pack or gather it and tie with some string or a rubber band to create a handle whatever you prefer as long as the ingredients stay inside the cloth.
- Place on the affected area for 20 minutes.

9. Tinctures

Ingredients

- For fresh herbs
- 1 oz fresh chopped herb to 2 oz of 95% alcohol
- For dried herbs
- 1 oz dried herb to 5 oz of 40% alcohol

Instructions

- Fill a glass jar with herbs without packing them down. Add alcohol to the jar and put the lid on the jar.
- Shake well and store the jar in a cool dark place, shaking the jar daily, for 4 to 6 weeks.

- ❖ Strain through a cheesecloth, squeezing the herbs to extract as much liquid as possible.
- ❖ Store the tincture in a glass jar in a dark place. Never leave your tincture in sunlight.

Ingredients

- ❖ dried herbs single or multiple
- ❖ vodka 80 proof or more (preferably 100 proof)

Instructions

- ❖ Put herbs in a quart-size Mason jar to about 1/2 full (not packed down).
- ❖ Pour a bit of boiling water over the herbs to help release nutrients (optional).
- ❖ Pour vodka overall to fill the jar to just below the bands.
- ❖ Cover the jar. Tip upside down a few times to wet all the herbs with the vodka.
- ❖ Put in a cool, dark location for 4 to 6 weeks. Each day during this time, tip the jar upside down a few times.
- ❖ After steeping for 4 to 6 weeks, strain. Discard herbs (compost) and put the extract in a jar(s) or 4-ounce dropper bottles.
- ❖ Store in a cool and dark location. Keeps a long time.
- ❖ Airtight, sterilized glass containers

- Enough chopped fresh herbs to fill each container halfway
- Dried herbs can be used instead to make more concentrated herbal tinctures
- High proof vodka. Everclear can also be used if it is legally available for purchase in your locale.
- Cheesecloth or a fine grade strainer

Instructions

- Chop your fresh herbs so that they naturally begin to release their aromatic oils.
- Place your herbs in each container using the measuring guidelines shown above.
- Fill with alcohol. Allow enough room at the top to ensure that there is room for the alcohol and herbs to mix well when shaken.
- Store in a cool, dry, dark area. Shake each container at least once per day for 30 days. Strain the tincture with layered cheesecloth or a fine grade strainer.

To Make An Herbal Infusion, You Will Need Three Things:

- 1 tablespoon dried herb of your choice
- 1 cup boiling water
- Glass jar with a tight lid (make sure it is very clean)

- ❖ The quantities of herbs and water can be increased proportionately to make a larger infusion if you wish. If you want to make 1 quart at a time, for example, this will require about 1 cup of dried herb and 1 quart of water. However, it's best to start with a small volume on your first infusion of any herb to avoid waste if you find you don't like it.
- ❖ While making the infusion, be sure to keep the jar covered at all times to contain the steam. The heat that's trapped inside is crucial to releasing those beneficial compounds in the herbs.
- ❖ Place the herbs in a glass container.
- ❖ Pour boiling water over the herbs so they are completely covered.
- ❖ Seal the jar with a tight-fitting lid to keep the steam and volatile oils from escaping.
- ❖ Allow the infusion to steep until the water cools to room temperature or for the time recommended by the infusion recipe. In general, roots and barks require the longest infusion (or a decoction) of about 8 hours. Leaves should be infused for a minimum of 4 hours, flowers for 2 hours, and seeds and fresh berries for at least 30 minutes.
- ❖ Strain the spent herbs out of the water using cheesecloth or a fine-mesh strainer (or both). Repeat if necessary to remove all of the herbs.

❖ The resulting liquid is called an infusion. Clean out the jar and pour the infusion back into it for storage. An infusion can be refrigerated for up to 48 hours. After this, it should be discarded.

CHAPTER 4: HERBAL REMEDIES FOR YOUR CHILD

0-2 Month

1. Newborn Dill [Anethum Graveolens]

Baby Dill is an aromatic herb, botanically classified as Anethum graveolens. The herb is a member of the Umbelliferae family, also known as the celery, carrot, or parsley family, and is cultivated for its delicate fresh leaves. Baby Dill is harvested at the very early stages of growth when the plant is still small and tender, and the flavor is milder. Though the herb is most often associated with pickling, Baby Dill is also popular in Scandinavian, Eastern European, Indian and Mediterranean cuisines.

Nutritional Value

Baby Dill is a great source of vitamins A and C and a good source of manganese, iron, and folate. The herb also contains calcium, riboflavin, niacin, and potassium and trace amounts of vitamin

B6, dietary fiber, magnesium, phosphorus, zinc, and copper. Its medicinal properties are due to the presence of monoterpene compounds, flavonoids, volatile oils, and amino acids. Dill has also demonstrated antibacterial properties.

Applications

Baby Dill is most often used fresh, but it is also used in its dried, or dehydrated, form. It may be used in fresh or cooked preparations, or as a garnish. It is often paired with fish, especially salmon, and in cream or wine-based sauces. Pair Baby Dill with yogurt, soft cheeses or cream, cucumbers, lentils, tomatoes, dried fruit, seafood, poultry, and beans. Use it as a salad herb or in pasta dishes with smoked fish or caviar, or in barley, quinoa, couscous, or bulgur wheat dishes. In Greek, Turkish and Slavic cuisine the herb is paired with chicken, spinach, mushrooms, and lamb. In Germany, it is paired with eggs, cheese, and potatoes. Keep Baby Dill dry until ready to use. If it becomes wilted, you can put the stems in a glass of water and cover it with a plastic bag. Baby Dill will keep refrigerated for up to a week and it can be frozen and kept for up to 2 months.

Recipe For Dill For Newborns Is As Follows:

- ❖ Pour a teaspoon of shredded fennel blooms over a glass (200ml) of hot water and put in a water bath to cook for 40 minutes.

- ❖ Pour the finished brew into a bottle.
- ❖ Leave to cool at room temperature.
- ❖ Fennel has similar properties, but they are more marked. If you like, prepare a remedy for fennel colic. This can be done as follows:
- ❖ Take a teaspoon of fennel seeds and a glass (200ml) of water for a daily dose.
- ❖ Pour the seeds with boiling water.
- ❖ After 1-1.5 hours, drain the infusion through the gauze and leave it to cool.

2. Lavender (Lavandula angustifolia)

You want the absolute best for your little one. You want to help them sleep well; feel better quickly if they get sick, and stop any pain or discomfort. Most of all, you want them to be happy and content. And you want to do it using a safe natural remedy.

Enter lavender essential oil. Just one whiff of lavender can immediately make your kid (and you) feel calm and more relaxed. It's the most widely used essential oil to ensure a good night's sleep for your baby or child. But its aromatherapy benefits don't stop there. It's also a great pain reliever, can help with colic and skin rashes, ease a fever and congestion, and naturally boost your child's mood and emotions. Most importantly, it's kid-safe.

One study found that mothers that bathed their infants in lavender-scented water experienced multiple benefits for both mom and baby. Mothers became more relaxed and touched and smiled at their babies more often. Their babies, in turn, looked at their mothers more, cried less often, and spent more time in deep sleep after bath-time.

It's also been found that a lavender oil massage can also help relax a fussy baby and encourage longer and deeper sleep. After introducing a bedtime massage routine with mothers and their babies, a study found that bedtime becomes easier, and the babies experienced less night-time waking.

As lavender essential oil quickly and safely relaxes the body and calms the mind, it can also be a life savior if your little one is anxious, insecure, or in any form of emotional distress - helping to soothe that incessant crying that can be so stressful for any mother.

Lavender is soothing and non-toxic, making it a favorite for babies not less than 2 months of age. In addition to being a natural antiseptic, lavender is also naturally sedative and its calming effects can alleviate muscle pains. To use, dilute lavender at a ratio of up to .5 percent and massage the blend along the baby's jawline.

3. Roman Chamomile

Roman Chamomile is one of the safest essential oils, and you can use it with very young babies (as young as zero to two months). At birth, the baby's digestive system is not fully developed yet. It is therefore common that during his first months of life, your baby experience digestive disorders such as colic, gas, bloating, or constipation. Chamomile is effective to relieve these issues and promote digestion in children thanks to its antispasmodic, anti-inflammatory, and soothing properties.

Benefits

Soothe Skin Irritation

Chamomile helps soothe irritated skin, redness, itching, and common skin conditions in infants. It has soothing and anti-inflammatory properties thanks to its rich concentration of flavonoids and is perfectly suited to the sensitive skin of babies. To soothe the baby's skin, you can use chamomile in different forms: hydrosol, floral water, essential oil, or herbal tea.

To Calm The Itching:

Pour 2 to 3 tablespoons of chamomile hydrosol into the baby's bathwater. If you do not have a hydrosol, you can make a cup of chamomile tea and mix it with the baby bathwater.

To Relieve Irritation And Redness:

Apply chamomile hydrosol or floral water to a sterilized compress. Apply it on the irritated area (previously cleaned and dried) 2 to 3 times a day. You can also put chamomile hydrosol and floral water in a spray bottle and apply it to the irritated skin.

Promote Sleep And Reduce Anxiety

All parents know it well: from your baby's birth, you are very unlikely to have an uninterrupted night. Although babies' sleep cycles evolve over the months, sleep disorders are common among infants and can have various causes: anxiety, toothache, fear of darkness, nightmares, etc. ... Chamomile helps calm the nervous agitation in baby, relax and improve sleep quality.

Before Putting Baby To Bed:

Give her a few teaspoons of chamomile tea diluted with a little water before bedtime.

You can also give her/him a relaxing massage with 1 drop of the essential oil of noble chamomile (Chamaemelum Nobile) diluted in a teaspoon of sweet almond oil. Not only will it help your little one relax and fall asleep serenely, but it will also strengthen your bond.

Calm Eye Irritation

Chamomile can be used in infants with conjunctivitis and eye irritation. It is effective in decongesting the eyes and calming the inflammation of conjunctivitis that causes itchy eyes. Its use is very simple and safe for babies. Just clean the eyes several times a day with chamomile tea, and after a few days, conjunctival symptoms and eye irritation will fade.

To Soothe Conjunctivitis:

Apply cooled chamomile tea on a compress. Clean the baby's eyes with the soaked compress by emphasizing the corners of the eyes and eyelashes. Soak a new compress of chamomile tea and apply it gently on the eyelids for 1 to 2 minutes. Repeat 4 to 5 times a day (or more) to help fight off the infection.

4. Astragalus

Like many safe herbs for infants, astragalus is known to boost the function of the immune system, thereby strengthening an infant's resistance to catching diseases. It is known to prevent children from contracting any illness or disease and also strengthening the immune system of a child after a disease.

How To Use

Add a slice of the root to a cup of water to make tea, or add it to stews, soups, or even to your pot of rice. The root itself should not be consumed, but it will release its beneficial properties in the boiling process.

2-12 Months

1. *Geranium*

Geranium essential oil is derived from steam distillation of the leaves of Pelargonium graveolens, a plant species native to South Africa. The geranium essential oil can be diluted with a carrier oil, such as sesame oil, and used topically on the skin. You can use it as a spot treatment for acne or itchy skin, or as a massage oil.

Some carrier oils may cause an allergic reaction when applied to the skin. Before using, do a patch test on a small area to make sure it doesn't cause a reaction. When diluting essential oils with a carrier oil, it's important to follow these dilution guidelines for one-two months to the one-year-old baby; 3 to 6 drops of essential oil per 6 teaspoons of carrier oil is a safe amount.

How To Make Geranium Oil At Home

If you have several weeks to spare, you can make geranium oil at home:

- ❖ Snip about 12 ounces of rose geranium leaves off the plant.
- ❖ Fill a small, clear glass jar around halfway up with olive or sesame oil and submerge the leaves, covering them completely.
- ❖ Seal the jar tightly and place it on a sunny windowsill for a week.

- ❖ Strain the oil through a cheesecloth into a different glass jar. Leave the geranium leaves behind.
- ❖ Add a supply of fresh geranium leaves into the oil.
- ❖ Seal the new jar and again leave it on a sunny windowsill for one week.
- ❖ Continue these steps each week for an additional three weeks (total of five weeks).
- ❖ Pour the essential oil into a bottle that can be kept tightly closed. Keep it in a cool, dry place, and use it within one year.

2. Mandarin (Citrus Reticulata) –Promoting Sleep.

Mandarin has calming effects similar to lavender, making it a great nighttime alternative for babies who are allergic to the scent of lavender. The sweet scent of mandarin is favorable to other orange varieties because it's not phototoxic. This means that even when diluted and applied directly to the skin, it shouldn't cause skin irritation.

3. Eucalyptus globulus

Eucalyptus oil is an extract from the leaves of the eucalyptus tree. The oil has a composition of more than 100 different compounds. Single distilled eucalyptus oil, which is crude oil, may contain more compounds in different quantities than the double-distilled eucalyptus oil, which is rectified. For instance, eucalyptus globulus oil has nearly 60% cineole and 40% other compounds. Following rectification, the oil contains 80% cineole and 20% other compounds.

Eucalyptus oil, one such essential oil, is said to have antibacterial and antiseptic action. The oil is used for these healing properties and has been in use as a popular home remedy for thousands of years. It is used as a therapy to treat respiratory problems such as cold, bronchitis, cough, and pneumonia in some cultures.

Eucalyptus is a natural expectorant that can help unclog respiratory congestion as it possesses antiseptic and antibacterial properties, making it a favorite during the cold winter months. Eucalyptus oil is used as a natural therapy to treat pneumonia, bronchitis, coughs, colds, and other respiratory ailments. It helps strengthen the immune system as well by improving respiratory circulation and providing antioxidant benefits. Cineole – more commonly known as camphor – is an organic compound present in eucalyptus oil that can help reduce pain and inflammation.

The type of eucalyptus species you buy for your baby is critical. When using Eucalyptus essential oil to treat congestion, parents should only use Eucalyptus Radiata for their children and infants. Eucalyptus Radiata contains a lower content of cineole than the widely available Eucalyptus Globulus and can, therefore, when diffused, be used with babies. While Eucalyptus globulus is safe for adults, it should not be used on children under the age of two. Eucalyptus Globulus contains a high content of cineole which is too harsh for the babies and can cause central nervous system and breathing problems. Eucalyptus Globulus should not be "applied to or near the faces of" or "otherwise inhaled by" children under one year of age.

4. Tea Tree (Melaleuca Alternifolia) –Reducing Germs

The botanical name of the tea tree, which is native to Australia, is 'Melaleuca alternifolia'. It is the source of tea tree oil. The leaves and twigs of it are treated with a steam and distillation process to obtain the medicinal oil. The oil has medicinal and disinfectant properties. Tea tree is a natural antimicrobial, antifungal, and disinfectant. Adding a few drops of tea tree oil to an unscented oil can help with diaper rash and fungal infections. Tea tree is a stronger oil that can be harsh on the skin, so it should be avoided on babies younger than six months old and carefully patch-tested on older infants.

Benefits Of Tea Tree Oil For Infants

The tea tree oil has several health benefits, which makes it a herbal remedy you need to have at your disposal. Mentioned below are some of the benefits of this oil.

1. Cures Skin Infections.

This oil is a natural antibacterial and antiseptic. It can be used to treat topical skin infections in babies and children. It is highly effective against wounds, insect bites, diaper rashes, and more.

2. It Helps Heal Wounds Faster.

When applied to injuries, the oil's antibacterial nature kills bacteria that are present on wounds and helps them recover more quickly. The oil can also reduce scarring of skin after a wound heals or in cases such as chickenpox blisters.

3. Treats Fungal Infections.

The tea tree oil for baby skin is highly effective in treating fungal infections such as ringworm in babies as it has a powerful anti-fungal effect. It also kills several harmful microbes in the protozoan family that can cause skin infections, rashes, and disease.

4. Strengthens The Immune System.

When you apply tea tree oil to the skin, it strengthens your immune system and helps build resistance to diseases. It does so by having a stimulating effect on hormone secretion and blood circulation. Due to this, your baby will be less prone to infections.

5. Cures Cough And Cold.

The tea tree oil for baby cold and cough is an excellent remedy to ease your baby's respiratory congestion. Since the oil has expectorant properties, it has been used for a long time to treat cold and cough. The treatment is as simple as rubbing oil on the baby's chest and throat to provide relief from a cough.

6. Improves Blood Circulation.

The anti-inflammatory properties of this oil help ease the pain in the body. Rub this oil on the muscles of your baby and he will feel better. The oil also reduces inflammation and improves blood circulation when applied over sore muscles. This promotes faster recovery.

7. Keeps The Skin Healthy.

The oil enables sweating which in turn helps your baby's skin to expel waste and other toxic substances that may have accumulated over time. This helps in keeping the baby's skin healthy.

8. Promotes Good Health.

Adding a few drops of tea tree oil to your baby's bathwater can promote good health. Its balsamic properties boost a baby's overall health.

How To Use Tea Tree Oil On Baby

Tea tree oil is available in the concentrated form as an essential oil. It should never be applied directly to the baby's skin. Mix it with a carrier oil such as olive oil, sweet almond, or coconut oils to dilute it, and then use it on your baby.

12 Months-5 Years

1. *Palmarosa [Cymnopogon martinii]*

Naturally balancing for the skin and emotions, palmarosa blends well with bergamot, cedarwood, and geranium. With a beautiful fresh, green, and floral scent, this soothing organic oil is steam distilled from the wild-growing grass near Tororo, in eastern Uganda. We've worked with a young farmer, Joel, to set up the distillery for aromatic crops grown on local farms, creating valuable employment.

Key Action: Cleansing

Latin Name: Cymbopogon martini

Country Of Origin: Uganda

Blends Beautifully With: bergamot, cedarwood, and geranium

Ingredients: Cymbopogon Martini Oil

Range: Essential Oils

Directions

1. Bath & Shower

Inhale the aromatic stream while your skin absorbs all the benefits of the oil. For adults, add up to 5 drops in 2 tbsp bath oil, shower gel, full-fat milk, or carrier oil. For children over 2 years old or adults with sensitive skin, reduce the amount to up to 2 drops per 2 tbsp.

2. Inhalation

This technique helps to clear your head and nose. For adults, add 4–6 drops to a bowl of steaming water, place a towel over your head and breathe. Children over 2 years old, adults with sensitive skin, and asthmatics should not inhale directly. Instead, place the bowl of hot water with added oils in the room nearby.

3. Massages

Balances your body and mind while helping to ease aching muscles. For adults, use up to 7 drops in 1 tbsp of base oil. For children over 2 years old or adults with sensitive skin, use up to 3 drops in 1 tbsp of base oil.

4. Diffusers & Burners

A natural air freshener, this technique creates a balancing ambiance and sets a mood. For adults, add 1–3 drops in a diffuser or burner. For children over 2 years old, add 1–3 drops in a diffuser.

Warning: Do not use undiluted on the skin. For external use only. Avoid contact with the eyes. Keep out of the reach of children. Flammable. Use within 12 months of opening.

5 years-12 years

1. Clary Sage [Salvia sclarea]

Clary sage (Salvia sclarea) is a flowering herb that's native to the Mediterranean Basin. The essential oil that's extracted from the leaves and buds of the plant has a clean, refreshing scent that you can use as a skin balm or gently inhale as part of an aromatherapy treatment

Clary sage is easy to grow in high-temperature areas. It's usually cultivated for its use as a flavoring in tea. It's also known by the names "clear eye" and "eyebright" because of its traditional use as a treatment for eye health. But it's now being studied for a variety of other health benefits.

Clary sage (Salvia sclarea) is traditionally used to boost confidence and self-esteem, as well as to improve mood. Studies show that clary sage has powerful antidepressant effects, and it seems to work by modulating dopamine and serotonin, brain chemicals linked with feelings of pleasure, happiness, and well-being. It may be even more effective when combined with ylang-ylang oil studies show that ylang-ylang can improve mood and boost self-esteem. Mix clary sage and ylang ylang essential oils in a diffuser in your child's room or combine in a spray bottle of water and spritz throughout your house. Sprinkle a few drops of clary sage on a cotton ball and inhale or sniff it right from the bottle. Or stir a few drops into a tub of warm water for a mood-lifting bath.

Ingredients

10 drops clary sage oil

Directions

Add 10 drops to an air diffuser or inhale directly from the bottle

2. Nutmeg [Myristica fragrans]

Nutmeg is the seed or ground spice of several species of the genus Myristica. Myristica fragrans (fragrant nutmeg or true nutmeg) is a dark-leaved evergreen tree cultivated for two spices derived from its fruit: nutmeg, from its seed, and mace, from the seed covering. It is also a commercial source of an essential oil and nutmeg butter. The California nutmeg, Torreya californica, has a seed of similar appearance, but is not closely related to Myristica fragans, and is not used as a spice.

Possible Benefits Of Nutmeg For Babies

Nutmeg contains several bioactive compounds possessing therapeutic properties. Its use is common in folk and alternative medicine to treat ailments and offer overall health benefits.

1. Relieve Indigestion: The use of nutmeg to treat digestive disorders is prevalent in traditional medicine. A freshly prepared decoction of nutmeg with honey is known to relieve gastrointestinal issues, such as indigestion. This decoction may be useful for babies older than 12 months who can consume honey.

2. Improve Appetite: Nutmeg has carminative effects, helping relieve flatulence, gas, and bloating . These effects may also help promote appetite in babies.

3. Support Immunity: Nutmeg has several bioactive compounds, such as eugenol, isoeugenol, and methoxyeugenol, with antioxidant properties. Besides, it has anti-inflammatory and immunomodulatory properties that may boost an infant's immunity in the long run

How To Use Nutmeg Or Jaifal In Babies

Take a grinding stone and wash it properly. Then pour some milk or water on it and rub the whole Nutmeg or Jaifal on the grinding stone in a circular motion and alternatively to and fro until you get some paste around 0.5 ml. Collect this paste in a spoon and pour some more milk or water to dilute it. Then give it to your baby directly post that feed her immediately to change the taste of the baby.

Dose: You can give around 0.5 ml of it one time during summers and two times during winters.

Precautions To Take While Feeding Nutmeg To Babies

- ❖ Before grating the whole nutmeg for use, wash it thoroughly under cold running water to remove dust and dirt that might be present on its surface.
- ❖ Grate the whole nutmeg to make its smooth paste, ensure no lumps or chunks are left.
- ❖ Every time you use ground nutmeg, rub a small amount of powder between your fingers and smell. If there is a faint aroma or no aroma, it usually signifies that the powder has become stale.
- ❖ Mix only a pinch or two of nutmeg paste or powder to a serving of baby food. Feeding nutmeg in excess can increase the risk of nutmeg intoxication (3).
- ❖ Preferably feed nutmeg with a food item that your baby is already consuming comfortably. It will help identify intolerance, sensitivity, or allergy towards nutmeg easily.
- ❖ If your baby looks uncomfortable after ingesting nutmeg, discontinue feeding and try again later.

- Nutmeg allergy is rare but possible. Consult a pediatrician before feeding nutmeg to the baby, especially if they have a family history of food and seed allergies.
- Keep the ground nutmeg away from your child's reach to avoid accidental ingestion.
- Nutmeg is a fragrant and flavorful spice with potential health benefits. You can use whole or ground nutmeg in minimal amounts to add flavor to your baby and toddler's foods. Purees, soups, stews, porridges, cereals, drinks, and baked goods are some recipes where nutmeg can go with other complementary herbs and spices.

CONCLUSION

Herbal medicine has its origins in ancient cultures. It involves the medicinal use of plants to treat disease and enhance general health and wellbeing. Some herbs have potent (powerful) ingredients and should be taken with the same level of caution as pharmaceutical medications. Many pharmaceutical medications are based on man-made versions of naturally occurring compounds found in plants. For instance, the heart medicine digitalis was derived from the foxglove plant. Herbal medicines contain active ingredients. The active ingredients of many herbal preparations are as yet unknown. Some pharmaceutical medications are based on a single active ingredient derived from a plant source. Practitioners of herbal medicine believe that an active ingredient can lose its impact or become less safe if used in isolation from the rest of the plant.

There is no question that physicians who spend more time with patients and listen more carefully will see benefits. Novella agreed that a caring, bonding practitioner is more likely to get patients to adopt healthier lifestyles and that these changes lead to better health. And he agrees that many patients do feel better when practitioners actively try to help them deal with vague, hard-to-diagnose complaints such as pain and fatigue, instead of telling them that there's no diagnosis or effective treatment.

But these aspects of a better patient-practitioner relationship should not be uniquely associated with alternative medicine, and such principles should not attempt to discredit the breakthroughs and innovations from the drug and device industry. Instead, we should look to our doctors to be the nurturing caregivers who take the time to listen to us, bond with us, and guide us toward healthier lifestyles and lower levels of stress.

Results: Many of the herbal products that are being given to children in the United States currently do not meet the standards of good manufacturing practices. No high-quality studies have been conducted to determine the efficacy of these products. Their concentrations of active ingredients are unpredictable, their labeling is inadequate, and they can cause toxicity.

Conclusions: The benefit-risk ratio of most herbal products remains unknown. Greater efforts and resources should be devoted to high-quality research to determine the effectiveness and tolerability of these widely used herbal products.

This review article presents important medicinal plants for the treatment and prevention of herbal remedies for the child.

These plants can be used for the preparation of new drugs; their active ingredients may also be used in the treatment of herbal remedies for the ld. In future studies, it is better to focus on the classification of herbal laxatives, based on their mechanisms for treating herbal remedies for the old.

Even in the light of the increased sophistication of modern healthcare as enriched by science and technology, the use of herbal medicine will continue to thrive in both poor and rich societies for many and probably different reasons. It is important for stakeholders: governments, farmers, scientists, healthcare providers (physicians, pharmacists, and nurses), and biotechnical engineers to give enough attention to herbal medicines and their challenges in a deliberate effort to create for it an appropriate niche that will ensure that it develops alongside with conventional medicine. The application of science and technology especially in the area of information resources, conservation and cultivation, production, analytical techniques, and quality control, clinical trials, and regulation should be promoted. These efforts will boost benefits, confidence, and safety in the use of HMs and its possible induction into mainstream healthcare. Though there are several pieces of literature on HM, this book nevertheless has stooped to collate in a simple, unambiguous, and readable manner a wide and indebt information that will be useful to all who have a stake in HM: scientist, healthcare professionals, engineers, and the general public.

Herbal remedies are commonly used by patients who access conventional health care. Few have been shown to have beneficial effects beyond those of conventionally regulated products, and they may be costly, adulterated with dangerous additives, inherently toxic, or cause the patient to forgo potentially curative care.

If a patient presents with a problem that might be due to an herb, the physician should discontinue the product and watch for resolution. If patients ask if "herbal medicines" in general are safe or effective, they should be counseled about the lack of regulations for quality, safety, or efficacy, the differences in preparations from different manufacturers, and the lack of a mechanism for reporting adverse effects. Curious patients can be directed to read the books mentioned, and cautioned against biased information that they may receive from health food store employees, pamphlets shelved near herbs, and the Internet.

www.ingramcontent.com/pod-product-compliance
Lightning Source LLC
Chambersburg PA
CBHW052356210526
45465CB00021B/36